Fit *and* Fabulous
from Fifty *Forward!*

Design the Fun Path That Suits YOU

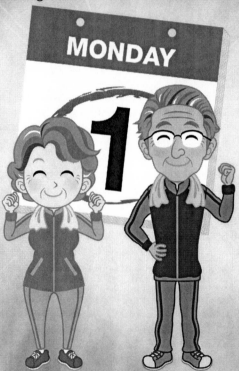

Barbara "Bobbie" Horowitz
The New 75 Year Old Kid on the Block.

BALBOA
PRESS
A DIVISION OF HAY HOUSE

Balboa Press books may be ordered through booksellers or by contacting:

Balboa Press
A Division of Hay House
1663 Liberty Drive
Bloomington, IN 47403
www.balboapress.com
1 (877) 407-4847

Because of the dynamic nature of the Internet, any web addresses or links contained in this book may have changed since publication and may no longer be valid. The views expressed in this work are solely those of the author and do not necessarily reflect the views of the publisher, and the publisher hereby disclaims any responsibility for them.

The author of this book does not dispense medical advice or prescribe the use of any technique as a form of treatment for physical, emotional, or medical problems without the advice of a physician, either directly or indirectly. The intent of the author is only to offer information of a general nature to help you in your quest for emotional and spiritual well-being. In the event you use any of the information in this book for yourself, which is your constitutional right, the author and the publisher assume no responsibility for your actions.

Any people depicted in stock imagery provided by Thinkstock are models, and such images are being used for illustrative purposes only. Certain stock imagery © Thinkstock.

Print information available on the last page.

ISBN: 978-1-5043-3770-0 (sc)
ISBN: 978-1-5043-3772-4 (hc)
ISBN: 978-1-5043-3771-7 (e)

Library of Congress Control Number: 2015912163

Balboa Press rev. date: 08/21/2015

Contents

Part III
Bobbie's Plan for Bobbie

Part IV
Unsolicited Recommendations and the Wrap-Up

Special Thanks To Two Spirits Who Live On as Inspirations

I thank my incredible baby sister, the late Susan Hank, whose spirit lives with me and encourages me every day. At the age of 19 Susie was operated on for what was diagnosed as Ileitis. The illness, Crohn's Disease, had not yet been discovered. She also learned that the blood transfusion given her during the surgery contained Hepatitis C. They had not yet learned to screen donated blood for this disease. Therefore, she lived each day aware that, at some point in her life, the Hepatitis would likely take hold of her. In spite of all she had to deal with, she managed to keep herself fit and in as good health as possible, She looked great and had a thriving career and her family, friends and former clients agree that she was a great contribution to all who knew her. Hepatitis may have taken her physically from us when she was 51 years old - but it couldn't take away her continuing to enrich us

I also thank my late spiritual coach, Barbara Van Diest, the woman to whom I dedicated my original book on the topic of fitness past 50. Without Barbara's tireless coaching I may never have believed I could be fit as I aged nor written any book on this topic. Barbara was beloved by many. Her TV show, "It's About You", which emanated from Tucson, inspired thousands. This is my post on her obituary in El Monte Ca. "Still with you every day, Barb. I feel you here with me too. I know it will be fine when I pass over to join you and I promise to keep living to my fullest while I'm still in this body. I know you're here."

Special thanks to a very physically alive member of the community

I thank my son, David F. Slone Esq., for his continuing support. I was born many years before computers and he is as brilliant in the field of technology as he is in entertainment and in law. He's loved in many entertainment communities in NYC and elsewhere and continues to promote his mom to them.

Dedication

I dedicate this book to the "Fit Fabulous You!" (The True You) who will reveal him/herself as a result of your reading "Fit & Fabulous From Fifty Forward!", at whatever age you may be.

Praise for Bobbie's Workshops

Bobbie named her workshops for the name she gave her plan to become fit when she was in her early 60s. She called her daily 'get to do's' "mini Qs". "The Find Your Mini-Qs workshops, that I recently attended were the first ray of hope I have found (after many attempts) in the losing weight/getting in shape battle. For the first time, no one was pushing hundreds of dollars of products I had to buy, nor solutions I couldn't possibly find the time, or motivation, to implement. Instead, I was encouraged to find my own path and chart a course to success that I developed (with guidance, of course). For me, this meant creating a phased approach using terminology and methods that I fully understood and supported. As someone who directs shows and provides professional corporate training and consulting services, I could easily relate to the teaching methodologies being presented here. I highly recommend everyone struggling with weight issues to 'find their Q'! It has sure helped me!"

—Tom Stajmiger, Performance Director,
Corporate Consultant/Trainer

"I found working with Bobbie inspiring, and I got in touch with some deep-seated patterns inside, which help me to unload a lot of the heaviness I felt. So I was able to lighten up physically as well. Finding my Q has led me to even more rewarding experiences as a lyricist. We are close to finishing a new musical called *Bollywood and Vine*, based on a movie of the same name: book by Edward Jordon, music by Daniel Neiden. We've had a great year with our family show *Rapunzarella White*. This month I began work on two more musicals. Check my website for updates. www.bosomoonproductions.com. Take a Q from me ... it's a high 'Q'uality way to live. Thank you, Bobbie."

—June Ospa, Playwright, Theater Coach

"Bobbie is one of the most inspirational people I have met in a very long time. After taking her workshop, I not only lost thirty pounds (yay!) However, I was also inspired to write a new cabaret act. I am really excited about my life again. All those baby steps and small, short-term goals really add up to major changes. Keep up the good work, Bobbie!"

—Diana LeBlanc, Singer, Legal Assistant

"I have known Bobbie for a long time. She is an outstanding individual with a huge intellect. Plus, she is not afraid to think creatively! I wanted to experience her workshop to gain advice for building my own 'sports prof' personal brand, my sports textbook, and my sports education company ... Sports Career Training LLC. Her insights and comments helped me crystallize my star and increase my own productivity. It was stimulating!"

—Frank E. Cuzzi, M.B.A..ports Prof—
The Complete Sports Manager

"Thank you so much for your ongoing generosity and for allowing me to learn and gain from you each time I'm in your presence. I continue to learn so much from you and am constantly inspired by the incredible gifts you offer every time I'm lucky enough to be with you ... My best wishes to you for another amazing and successful chapter as your new book inspires all of us to be healthy, wealthy, and wow!"

—Richard Skipper, Press Representative/MC/Coach/Producer

Introduction

The star you truly are is right here!
Let it shine!
Most importantly, **have faith in yourself.**
You can do this! Plus, have *fun* doing it!

As you read this book, you'll learn to design your own path to allow the slimmest, strongest, sexiest possible you shine out - and you'll give your path a name that's *fun* for you to say and think about.

When I was sixty, I had to drop over thirty-five pounds, handle a very high cholesterol count, a severe case of osteoarthritis and find clothing that would look good on my now enlarged frame! I'd gained weight and lost fitness between ages fifty-five and sixty. I was working intensely on a theatrical project I loved, which was excellent for me. However, I was eating and moving according to someone else's needs rather than according to my body's needs.

Hint: Give the path you design for yourself a name that makes you smile—or even better, giggle! I repeat this often because I've found that having fun is likely to keep people on track. We'll have whole chapter on naming your path.

I call my path My Mini-Qs. "Mini-Qs" stands for the minimum quantity of various activities I undertake to reach my goals of being slim, strong, and sexy. I *get to do* most of them daily. Some are weekly, and some are monthly. You'll be able to follow the path you design for yourself, to peel away everything that isn't that star you really are.

Maybe you're saying, "She calls them Mini-Qs? What—is she nuts?"

Believe me, I would have thought the same thing about that name. However, if a lucky thought hadn't come into my head—a thought that led me to choose that name for my plan—I wouldn't have peeled away the part of me that was out of shape and not feeling well. The name helped keep me doing ... *drum roll* ... my *minimum quantity* of daily, weekly, or monthly tasks I needed to do in order to accomplish my goals.

This will be discussed further in Chapter 5.

I wanted to find a word that wasn't the norm. I, also, didn't want to use a word that brought forth negative feelings. . I wanted to find words that aren't associated with dull routine.

After the book *The 7 Habits of Highly Successful People* by Stephen Covey was published, the word "habit" took on a more positive connotation. We can get bogged down in semantics; but as you become and stay as fit, strong, and healthy as you possibly can be you will get in the habit of following routines. I was able to shift my thinking about "routine" and turn it into something fun! You can do this too!

For some reason, "routine" and "dull" have become synonymous in our culture. The word "mini-quota" came to equal the least number of times I would do something each day and the different things I would eat each day to get a result. The words literally popped into my head. At the beginning, while I was using the phrase, I didn't even realize that mini-quota was the phrase I was looking for. I could set the mini-quota of things to do each day so I could reach it. I could then increase any of my daily mini-quotas that were too easy to complete, or I could lower any that were not getting done because they were too difficult.

Most of the "diets" I'd heard of had to do with denying myself and knowing what I shouldn't do. I started using just the letter Q because "quota" suggests *having* to do something. Instead, it's about *getting to do something* that leads us to what we want, which has a positive connotation. In addition, with mini-Q, I concentrate on *doing* my Qs rather than on *not doing* something.

I didn't have "No more ice cream, Bobbie!" running around in my head. Instead, my head was holding "Time for that apple!"

I'm thrilled that I discovered I could design my very own path to reach my goals, a path that totally suited my particular body and personality. This allowed me to get my body (and spirit) into shape and keep it in shape and enjoy the process!

I put two and two together and designed my path to body rejuvenation when I was in my early sixties. That was over a decade ago! I've been in shape and loving it ever since! I certainly didn't do it totally on my own. I researched and asked questions and got helpful ideas, and I stumbled upon some great ideas. I absorbed the ideas that were given to me and then put them together in my mind in a way that helped me use them to carry out my plan.

By the way, I didn't make up the concept of peeling away everything that wasn't my true star-self. I give credit for that to one of the greatest artists in history, Michelangelo.

When asked how he sculpted the magnificent marble statue of David, Michelangelo di Lodovico Buonarroti Simoni is said to have replied, "I took the stone and merely chipped away all that wasn't David."

Guess what?
I'll repeat! You can - and should – revise your plan when needed.

If a movement or a particular food choice you made seems yucky to you or doesn't seem to be working for you, you can keep revising it until it works for you.

You can even up your mini-Q! I've found I can almost double my possible walking quota! Yesterday was what most people were calling "frigid." Can you believe that I actually enjoyed walking a little over eighty blocks! These are Manhattan uptown/downtown blocks. This distance measures four miles for the day, as compared with my previous mini-Q of a mile and a half (thirty blocks).

I've learned to keep revising, both when I can do more and when I need to cut down on activity and I can add or subtract certain foods from my daily intake.

Before we go ahead, I advise you to make it a point to keep up with the latest studies pertaining to health and to revise accordingly. Scientists and doctors are constantly learning new things about our bodies. Thankfully, this has been an area of constant discovery.

You'll also find that I often repeat things in this book. I do this on purpose. While great writing is supposed to be carefully laid out without needing repetition, I found that I needed to repeat ideas to myself as I went through the first several months of the process of getting into my true shape. It was the only way I could incorporate my "ah-ha moments" into my daily life.

The method of devising your strategy will remain the same. The actual items within that strategy may change as you learn more about your body and what's available to you to help it flourish.

Are you ready to be as fit and strong and sexy as you possibly can be?

Then let's get started!

PART I
Revealing the Winner in You

CHAPTER 1

Do You Think You Are a Winner Right Now?

If you're like most people, your deep-down answer is "NO".

I was curious to find out if I was the only person who had ever thought of suicide. Granted, only a couple of times have I thought things would be easier if I were dead. However, people usually say that I'm a positive person. So if I could have a thought like that, I suspected that I wasn't the only one.

This may sound extreme, but just before I wrote the first edition of this book, I asked more than 125 people, who appeared to be over fifty years of age, "Did you ever think of killing yourself?" I asked people who looked as though they were in shape and people who did not. Can you believe that only one person out of all those I asked said they'd never ever given a moment's thought to suicide? I don't know the name of the man who said he'd never thought of it; (I purposely did not ask people their names). These were people I met on busses and subways or while walking on the street (in NYC most people travel by public transportation and I'm always meeting new people on, or while waiting for, busses and subways or just walking on the street.)

If you're thinking: *"Bobbie Horowitz is crazy! I'm in great shape. I'm fabulous looking! I'm sexy! I'm smart and I've done everything I ever dreamed of doing with my life!"*- I take my hat off to you and say, "Bravo!" I cheer you because I know you're right – and - I'd advise you to read this book to give you a plan of action in case future issues come up for you. Then give the book to your friends. You know which friends: the friends who complain that they're too fat/skinny/mushy/tired/headachy, getting old—you name it!

I was in my mid-sixties before I fully realized my mission in life. My mission is to see that you totally love yourself—and I take responsibility for doing all that's in my power to have that happen. There are very few people who need no help in this area.

In this book, I concentrate on your physical being. I wrote this book:

1. To open your heart to what a divine, human work of art you are and
2. To open your mind - so you can allow yourself to bring the divine, physical you to the fore. My goal is for you to design a pleasurable, doable way to improve what you can about your physical being. I also want you to learn how to accept what you can't improve until you find a way to improve it, so you can love every bit of you. I'll contend that you are an awesome work of art and that you don't have to change yourself! You just need to let that work of art that you are come out from under its coverings. The coverings may be extra pounds, flab, or malfunctions you can avoid.

This book is not about changing your true self. However, you will change your appearance. If you're flabby, too skinny, etc., you're not showing your true self. You'll learn how to choose actions—thought out specifically for you and your lifestyle. I call my actions

4

mini-Qs. When you use (whatever you've named yours) daily, you'll dust away the need to choose the actions that have buried *you the artwork* and created clouds around *you the star.*

What we each need to focus on is how to choose actions that will bring out the wonderful, unique creations we are and how to clean off the *schmutz* (Yiddish for "dirt") that's been added. This may be easier said than done. Sometimes we don't realize we're choosing actions that are not based on the truth; rather, our actions are based on erroneous thoughts we've come to believe are true.

In this book, I take on the responsibility of doing everything I can to help you scrape away all that isn't you, physically. This step will take some mental scraping, but it's worth the effort.

I have an inner knowing that Earth is heading toward the day when each human accepts the fact that he or she is wonderful, when people won't fear "the other guy," and feel they need to protect themselves from "the other guy". I'm jubilant when I think of it because, even though you and I will probably not see this happen in our physical lifetimes - this goal isn't impossible!

Things happen. How we react to them is our choice. It's been said in different ways thousands of times. I'm repeating what so many others have said because I'm still in the process of incorporating these discoveries into my own being.

Last month (May 2015) I celebrated my seventy-fifth birthday. It was, indeed, a celebration! The first edition of this book was published shortly after I celebrated my seventieth birthday. One of my goals is to keep expanding this knowledge and incorporating it into my brain and body for as long as I'm alive. When I say incorporate, I mean not just mentally understand the knowledge but also live as if it is so.

Several people will need to hear the ideas I'm sharing many times before they can incorporate them. <u>If you get these ideas in one take, please forgive me for repeating them. Some people need to read them many times.</u>

CHAPTER 2

Seven Ways We May Be Hiding Our Star to Keep It from Shining

I believe we hide due to **FEAR**. It can be scary to be out there as a star. You may not have expected that sentence. However - look what success often brings! People expect great things from you and you become more visible. This can be daunting, either consciously or unconsciously.

I've been scared of the spotlight. I'm not a psychologist, but I've spoken with several, and I've read many books that cover this topic. I'll bet you have too.

Remember that you are that star. You're that star, whether or not it is yet shining to its full potential. We'll find out what's blocking it's light. Take a deep breath and accept yourself as you are now. Love and accept yourself every step of the way. Allow yourself to be patient during the process, which, by the way, may move more quickly than you've imagined it would. If it doesn't move quickly, you can still love yourself and revise your path.

The following are some of the ways you may have been hiding your star.

1. *Playing dumb.* When we play dumb, we make believe that it doesn't matter if we look vital. What we're really making believe is that we don't matter. That pretense becomes reality.

2. *Avoiding pursuit of what we want.* We do this just to avoid a scary body sensation. Sounds silly, right? Of course, we are not aware we're doing this. Ask yourself questions when you're not making progress toward getting what you've hoped for. Ask yourself if your throat, stomach, or some other body part feels tight or if your skin is tingling. I've learned that bodily sensations caused by fear can stop me from making progress. By noticing these sensations and changing my thoughts about them, I can change my patterns. I learned this from David Friedman in his book *Thought Exchange.* For more information, see chapter 16.

3. *Finding reasons to put off regular doctor checkups.* I'm thankful that this was never a pattern in my family, and I never adopted this pattern. I know only a few people who avoid regular physical examinations. However, doctors have told me that quite a few people do fall into this pattern. I think that most people who don't go for checkups feel that they'll be looked upon as bad because they have not kept themselves from getting an illness or physical malfunction. I recommend that you get checkups for things that can be checked. You're not "bad boy or girl" for getting ill, but you are unwise for not having your body checked at regular intervals. It's much easier to cure most health problems when they are caught early. Then you can feel like the good boy or good girl you are.

4. *Dwelling on maladies or "handicaps" and not allowing them to go away.* I hear some people identify themselves by their

illnesses, and some people won't listen to information about possible ways to cure an illness or at least mitigate its effects.

5. *Blaming weight or muscle problems on heredity.* While our genetic heritage may play a part—even a large part—in all our physical characteristics, that doesn't mean we can't be healthy or deal with many aspects of our physicality in ways that are different from our ancestors. In recent years, much has been discovered about dealing with various illnesses. My wonderful little sister, Sue Hank, would most likely be alive today if doctors had known to check blood for Hepatitis B before a transfusion. If this test, which became routine by 1990, had been available in 1965, my sister would probably be living today. She was a force who helped many people, so her life was extremely valuable. I can't help but think how many more people she could have helped in the eighteen years since her passing. I can't resist cheering Susie.

6. *Feeling we always need to please everyone.* This is a biggie! I confess that it continues to be a major issue for me to deal with. I address this issue in the next chapter and in other sections in the book. Let me give you an example. When people are dining out, many people feel they should eat what the rest of the group chooses. Underneath, they're frightened the group won't like them if they don't. I used to do this. I'm thankful I've learned that I help my friends more if I set a good example. If they can't take it, well, that's their problem. Your friends will respect you more when your star is shining in their eyes.

7. *Not getting physical exercise because belonging to a gym is too expensive and/or there isn't enough time.* Blaming our big midriff on a lack of time is like saying we don't deserve to get into shape. Everything else deserves the time but not our body. If you look hard to find a gym in your area that you can afford, you'll probably find one. If not, there are ways to exercise in life. We'll be talking more about this.

I remember discussing reasons why and ways in which we hide our greatness—in different areas of life—with my spiritual coach, the late Barbara Van Diest. In terms of looking as well as you can look and being as fit as you can be, you might wonder why there would be any fear attached. It's all good—right? It would seem so. However, issues can come up when you're a gorgeous teenager or adult or senior. Those of you who've been on either side of these feelings (feeling ugly or feeling "not liked" because you're too good looking) will understand what I'm speaking about. Pre-teen girls and boys can resent a beautiful or handsome member of their class or group because the good-looking young person gets positive attention for being good looking, and they don't. The same can be said for young people who are very bright or have great ability to get their points heard by authority figures, etc. The "who does he think he is" mentality can come into play.

I've come to believe that we wouldn't resent those who have great attributes we don't (think we) have if we hadn't been "taught" to resent those who have them. The people who "taught" you this probably had no idea this is what they were doing. Think about things you might have heard said about people at a dinner table or when leaving a party or a meeting, etc. I think that Oscar Hammerstein nailed this concept in his lyrics for the song, "You've Got To Be Taught", which was in the musical "South Pacific". (Wish I wrote that one!) The song teaches us that if we hate or fear or resent other people – it's because we were taught to.

I get moved every time I think of that song and it's truth.

While this may sound simplistic, if you think you're less fit and healthy or less good looking than might be possible for you to be, I urge you to sit quietly and think about your life as a child, as a teen, as a young adult, and see if any situations come to mind that may have painted a negative picture in your mind about you being number one in the area of fitness (or any other area of your life). About a year ago I enrolled in Nick Ortner's seven-week online tapping course for maximizing finances, and many of these "I'm not good enough" questions came up for me in that area.

You may also want to think about what you think would be demanded of you if you were at your best possible weight and strength. If you became one of the strongest and most facile people in your age group, would you be expected to look gorgeous every single day and to run to this and that event? In the back of your mind, does it seem like too much will be expected of you if you can't fall back on being too tired or being overweight or underweight or less than strong? I know it may sound strange to think that being at your best could cause problems and that NOT being at your best can make life easier for you - but I see this rearing it's head often for people I know and it may well come up—usually subconsciously—for you too.

It can look like a lot of work to get fit. I'm writing this book to show you that while there may be many to-dos (better to call them "get-to-dos") on the list you'll make for yourself, they'll all fit into your lifestyle and help your specific body and chemical makeup. When you can handle them with humor, it becomes your fun game. When you're the hottest, most energetic, youthful-looking fifty-, sixty-, seventy-, eighty-, ninety-year-old you can be, you will have the right to say no when people keep asking you to do things for them, things that don't benefit you—unless, of course, you truly want to do the specific things asked of you.

I'm still working on saying "No" myself. Learning to say "No" may take a while. I promise you, the time spent will be worth it. Pleasing people is wonderful—when it's serving you too.

CHAPTER 3

What Are <u>Your</u> Specific Reasons for Wanting to Be Fit?

It helps to have specific reasons. They help keep you going when you're feeling tired or frustrated.

It will help you if you have your answers to the following questions written down and in a place where you can easily find them. You'll be coming to pages in the book on which you'll actually write down the daily activities you'll undertake to reach your goals.

Grab a pad of paper and pen and write down your answers to the questions that follow.

Four Questions to Ask Yourself

It might seem as though the answers to the questions in this chapter are obvious. However, were it that simple, wouldn't everyone have done whatever they could to reach their optimum weight and stay as fit as they can be?

I think most people, at least subconsciously, are well aware of what fitness and a healthy lifestyle would do for them.

I applaud *you*! You're consciously going for it! You're coming for answers.

Every morning, think of the answers you write down. It'll help bring these questions to mind every day.

1. How will fitness and being my healthy weight help me?

I spoke with several people, some of whom are in great shape and others who say they want to get into great shape. Those who were in great shape simply listed what they thought of as their benefits from being healthy, and the others phrased their answers more like "wouldn't it be lovely if ..." Both groups listed just about the same things as benefits.

- *Less worry.* Wouldn't it be more enjoyable to spend less time worrying about health and more time feeling great about yourself? Being in shape will reduce the stress that comes from worry as well as the physical stress from carrying extra weight around with you.

- *More romance.* Just because you're fifty, sixty, seventy, eighty, years or older doesn't mean you can't have romance in your life! Romance can encourage a state of wellbeing. Granted, you needn't look like a calendar girl or boy to have love in your life. But it's much easier to feel romantic toward someone who feels good about him/herself. For those who aren't married, it usually helps to attract the opposite sex if you're in shape.

- *More stamina.* If you choose to—or need to—work, your life will be much easier if you have the energy to carry out your daily assignments. You can also turn these into Qs and watch your work improve and get noticed. You'll read more about this in a later chapter.

- *Increased ability to play.* Yes—play! Do you like to sing? Would you like to be a member of a theater group? Do you like to play sports? Would you love to travel? You'll be better. ble to enjoy all these activities and more.
- *Greater Longevity.* A Swedish study recently published in the *British Medical Journal* has given those who have reached or passed middle age hope and encouragement to begin a new, healthy lifestyle. The study discovered that starting a "solid exercise regime" after the age of fifty could raise one's level of longevity to that of those who have been exercising regularly all along. Note: When you design your Qs, you needn't refer to movement as a "regime"—you'll be getting the benefits of one anyway. The good news here is that *it's never too late to start.*
- *A more capable-looking and successful-looking appearance.* I thought this was interesting. One or two of the people I spoke with mentioned that there are people who can succeed and not allow being overweight to hold them back, as long as they have the energy to do their work and live their dreams. Having the energy is the kicker. This implies that it may take more to succeed when someone's out of shape, and some take on that task. I spend much of my time with people in the theatrical community. While all sizes and shapes of actors are needed to portray the population, there is certainly more work for people who are in good shape. Good health is also important because it will cost the production company, especially for film, big time if an actor, especially a leading actor, gets ill at the last minute.
- *Higher self-esteem.* (Note: when you feel great about yourself, my work is done!) When you feel great about yourself, you'll be able to listen to your intuition. You'll be able to trust the universe, which I've finally learned to do. But don't think I don't have to remind myself almost every day that I can have this trust!

2. How will being in shape and at my healthy weight help others?

This is a biggie!

We, very often, have more impetus to complete something if we know someone else, whom we care about deeply, is depending on us to achieve our goal. I was reading an article about a Bristol, England, taxi driver who wanted to use his weight loss to raise cash for cancer research. His wife was active in raising funds for cancer and Alzheimer's research.

- *A child.* Do you have a child? If you do, I'm sure I don't have to say much. I'm sure you'd give anything to benefit your child's welfare.
- *A grandchild.* A grandparent can be such joy for a little one. I can remember being with my grandparents as if it were yesterday. My dad's mother died of a heart attack when I was only six years old. She always had to stop every couple of minutes when we took walks. I try to avoid thoughts of my mother's mother through the long years of her illness. Her condition was somewhat due to the lack of medical knowledge at the time. However, I have a feeling healthier eating may have mitigated some of her suffering. Of course, then we didn't know about that, and we thought she was eating for good health. My mom's mom was the great cook in the family. She got dementia in her early fifties and then Alzheimer's. I don't know if they had the name for it yet. She died at about seventy-two. I think both of these women could have been my confidants for more years had we known more about healthy eating. I know that if you have grandchildren, you want to be there for them.
- *A husband or wife, boyfriend or girlfriend.* Do you have a spouse? If so, that person's life will be affected by you almost as much as yours will. If you're in great shape, you will worry less about becoming ill. You'll probably also be more relaxed

when you feel healthier and stronger and you feel you look terrific in clothes that fit you.

- *An aging parent.* How lucky you are if you have a living parent. If you do, your parent needs you on two levels. First, your parent may need your help with different living arrangements, with organizing his or her possessions, and with visiting other family members and friends. Second, and I think even more important, you parent's life will be enhanced by knowing that you're okay. You know how you feel about your children, if you have children.

I'm sure you can think of additional reasons for yourself.

3. Who else might need me to be fit?

- *Friends.* I know how I feel when friends of mine are ill. I get frustrated when I can't help them because they're not open to help. I'm so glad you are!
- *Business partners and clients.* If you're still working, your business partners and your customers need you to be vital and strong to help carry out the mission of your company. Since you bought this book and you're already interested in your well-being, I'm certain that your business or job truly serves the people who are your customers/clients.
- *Community associates.* When the body of a member of the theatrical or cabaret community begins to fail, I feel my heart sink. You may belong to clubs, charitable groups, alumni groups, etc. Certainly our bodies will someday leave the planet. I do think the choices we make can affect the time we're "supposed" to leave. I repeat—I want you to stick around!
8. *People who are involved in or benefit from my projects— projects that I'm passionate about!* Passion may be the strongest

motivation of all. I told my dear friend, the beloved Sidney Myer, who books *Don't Tell Mama!*—a NY cabaret, to book a date for me to do a show in May 2048! You know why I did that? It means I'll have to show up! (I'm hoping Sidney will be there too!)

I'm certain that you can add to this list. The important thing for you to know is that people are counting on you, even if it's only for their happiness—and yours.

Note—if you happen to be a teen or in your twenties, and you're reading this book, (which, by the way, can help YOU get fit too) please do the following:

1. Think about the stress your parents have when you're not well. They love you. Sometimes illness can't be avoided, but being fit certainly makes it less likely you'll get ill.
2. Think about your teachers, if you're still in school.
3. Think about your friends and neighbors.

4: I would love to help people I know. Can I help others get fit?

This is another biggie. Remember that helping others spurs us on.

- Look at the lists above. When you're in the shape you want to be in, don't be surprised if you find yourself starting to spread the word. People will start asking you how you did it.
- Some friends may say they desperately want to get in shape. They may complain about being fat or back pain since they "gained all that weight," etc. You may get excited and give them this book or tell them about what you're doing.

They may get excited and say they'll give it a try. They may actually see some progress with dropping pounds or having more energy. Then they might start complaining that they've put on weight, and you see them eating five pieces of cream cake when you go out to lunch with them. That day's lunch "mini-Q" for them has turned into five pieces of cream cake! So, you ask them what "Get To Do's" they've designed for themselves. They say, "I just can't think about that now. I had to have my floor repaired," or some such thing. I'll explain naming your tasks in more detail in Chapter. 4.

- If they didn't pay attention to you - it's not your fault. <u>You</u> needed to *want* to rejuvenate. So must they - to succeed.

CHAPTER 4

My Goals: Where Am I Going? Where Am I Now?

This is all about you! It's about finding what works best to bring out the best you. I've found that when people begin to allow themselves to be the physical star they truly are, as if by magic, they start coming into their own in all areas of their life. The more I observe and work with people, the more I understand that attaining what we want, in all aspects of our life, is based on the same principle and comes from the same source—what's going on inside our minds and how we handle our thoughts.

We often get stuck in our thoughts. You can always revise goals as you learn more about yourself.

Do you like to make lists? If you don't, then don't write out the lists! Filling them out isn't a requisite to dropping pounds or inches. Having a list for different aspects of getting fit in "Q Land" (As I call it. You can use the name you want to give it.) can be a great support. Lists can save you thinking time. If it reminds you of other plans you used to drop weight, and those were a pain in the neck—then don't fill out these lists. I do think it's a good idea for you to at least look at the lists and think about them. If you can know them well without writing anything, fine. Writing lists works for me. I find that the physical act of writing helps me remember the ideas I put down.

There's a list below for you to look at and fill out, if that works for you. Write down—or at least think of—the vision you have of your dream self (your true self). You may put your measurements in if you choose. It will be fun to see how close you come to reaching your dream measurements and weight and energy level and, for some people, even your height. Having good posture, if possible, can give you energy and boost your spirits.

If you haven't had a physical checkup in a while, this would be a good time to get one. If you haven't already asked your doctor to advise you on what would be an ideal weight or weight range for you, this would be a good time to do that (even if you have had a checkup this year).

When you put your list together, you'll have a basic vision (size and fitness) of yourself. *I found it very helpful to know that particular goals don't have to be written in stone. In some cases, they shouldn't be.* When you've reached your goals, you'll be the you that's left after you've chipped away what isn't you. Think of the statue of David. Michelangelo chipped the stone. The beauty of the mini-Q plan is that you can change your goals until you reach goals that best serve you.

Sometimes our goals themselves are based on false ideas we've been taught. For example, you might find you can weigh even less than you thought and still be very strong and healthy. You might see that you overestimated one or more of the changes and that it wouldn't really serve you to, for example, weigh as little as you originally put down. I know that when I was young, I had goals that were based on standards that society and the fashion magazines set up for me. They didn't produce the healthiest me.

While obesity is certainly a larger problem right now in terms of numbers affected, wanting to be skinny isn't healthy either. Years ago, I had a wonderful mother and daughter living in the apartment next to mine. The daughter was a beautiful young woman who needed to drop pounds but got addicted to starving and actually passed on as a result. I know that people our age are rarely affected by anorexia, yet I want to be clear that we're talking about healthy beauty.

Your Goal Sheet

Here is the Goal Sheet I used plus I've added some categories I didn't need to worry about, but that you might need to be concerned with. If these items have checked out well for you before you needn't add them.

Keep the month you're starting out in mind. Pick the month you've started reading the book. I'm putting down January 1st 2016 just as an example.

Goal Sheet for One Year From Today

1. On January 1, 2917 I shall weigh _____lbs.
2. On January 1, 2017 my waistline will measure _____inches
3. On January 1, 2017 my hips will measure _____inches
4. On January 1, 2017 my thighs will measure _____inches
5. On January 1, 2017 my breast (if you're male you might prefer chest) will measure _____inches
6. In January 1, 2017 my upper arms will measure_____
7. In January 1, 2017 my doctor will tell me that my cholesterol level is normal
8. In January 1, 2017 my heart rate will be normal (or will have improved to_____) Ask your doctor if you need to be concerned with this before you begin.
9. In January 1, 2017 my blood test will show no problems.

Note: For the medical questions you'll want to check the time for recovery with your doctor. I just made up the one-year approach. One year may not be right for you,

Note: You might want to fill out a goal sheet for your dental health too. Ask your dentist what you should be concerned with in regards to your mouth's health.

After you fill out your goals make out a duplicate list with the date you're beginning on it. In this second list, fill in where you are now. There's no good or bad place to start. It's just the block of stone you're in now. It's "all good".

If it gives you impetus to follow your "get-to-dos", you may want to make a file for your journey. You can have folders for food and for exercise.

If you wish, attach a full-length photo of you now in a folder and sign your name as "Hidden Star".

Hidden Star _____ now

(Your name goes on this line.)

Then, later, you can put in another full-length picture (date it) when you've uncovered the true you in terms of weight, etc.

Shining Star _____ revealed

(Your name goes on this line.)

You can attach index cards or a piece of paper and put down the figures for your height and weight and a brief description for body parts. You can measure your arms and thighs, etc. and put down the inches if that inspires you. Then just put a check next to certain items. For example, if you think you have dangling arms, chin, etc. This is for you to use as a future reminder of how much you've accomplished!

You can add any part of your body you notice: weight, height, general body description, muscles in arms, under-arm muscles, muscles in legs, thigh measurement, stomach muscles, hip measurement, waist measurement, back muscles, lines around eyes, puffiness under eyes, lines around mouth, lines on forehead, droopy neck, droopy jowls, puffy or hanging jaw line, spots on hands …

When you've written out your goals - write out your daily/ weekly "_____" (whatever you've named your tasks that will get you to reach your goals! As you know, I call my tasks my "mini-Qs" - i.e., the minimum quantity of each thing I have to do – or better said - "get to do" each day that will lead me to achieve my goal in any area. Saying I "get to do" it ups my spirit much more than if I use the terms "need to do" or "have to do". "Get to" sounds to me like I'm giving myself a gift.

This is a biggie! <u>Now that you've written down your goals and written down what you'll do on a daily basis to achieve these goals, put your goal sheet in a drawer and forget about it!</u>

Note: In part 2, we'll talk about checking your goal sheet every few months to see how far you've gotten and to see if you want to revise your daily activities. Then back in the drawer it will go!

Until you reach your goals, or have gotten close to reaching them. seeing them every day might not be encouraging to you because you haven't reached them yet.

Don't beat yourself up if it takes a little while to get into the momentum of just doing your _____ (your name for your daily tasks) every day. Keep clarifying them, and eventually you *will* get into it. We'll make the process fun too!

CHAPTER 5

Why Name Your Personal Path to Fitness?

This chapter should give you a better understanding of why I call my list of daily/weekly/monthly actions "mini-Qs".

As we discussed, <u>the name of the path you're now going to design—to chip away anything that isn't the strongest, healthiest, sexiest you possible—should put a smile in your heart and, if possible, give you a giggle!</u> Laughter is a great facilitator for positive activity.

My major purpose in using the letter Q to describe the plan is to camouflage previous stomach-tightening (in the nervous sense) ideas we've been carrying around for years. When you heard what "mini-Q "actually is, you probably laughed. I found I could camouflage the idea of "a plan" or a "routine" in such a way that my mind didn't make it a negative.

Camouflaging "Dull Routine"

"Everyone gets into a dull routine" is the first line of the song "Monotonous" from the musical revue, *New Faces of '52*. Eartha Kitt sang it to my enthralled ears. Do you remember that one?

I wanted to find a word that wasn't the norm—that wasn't associated with past failures, the times I shouldn't eat, what I shouldn't eat, etc. I wanted to get rid of the "shouldn't" part of it. *I wanted to find words that aren't associated with a "dull routine."*

For some reason "routine" and "dull" have become synonymous in our culture. *The word "mini-quota" came to mean the minimum times I would do something or the different things I would eat to get a result.* The word literally popped into my head. At the beginning, while I was using the phrase, I didn't even realize that mini-quota was the phrase I was looking for. I had a mini-quota of things to do each day. I set the mini-quota so I could reach it. I could then increase my mini-quota if it was too easy or lower it if it wasn't working as well as it could have. Then I started using just the letter Q because "quota" suggests *having* to do something. I changed the wording to *getting* to do something that leads us to what we want. With mini-Q, <u>I concentrated on *getting* to do my Qs rather than on *having to do* something.</u> I didn't have "No more ice cream, Bobbie!" running around in my head. Instead, my head was holding "Time for that apple!"

Many people I know feel stress when they're dieting. I want you to feel full and nourished and truly happy. That's why there's a whole chapter about letting go of stress. I feel happy because I feel strong and slim and great! I can also say I feel strong and slim and great because I feel happy! It works both ways. <u>You can choose to be happy before you begin your plan.</u> I'll talk about tapping in my unsolicited recommendations chapter. While Q does stand for quota, - and that can have negative connotations for some people - but with *"mini"* added in front of it, I was finding *the least amount of each activity needed to get the results* I wanted. Then I got to fit these into *my* lifestyle. The part that really works for me is that when I started saying "my mini- Q," it suddenly sounded funny. To my ear, "mini-Q" didn't sound like an obligation at all. It was the number of times I *got* to do something. Yay!

To repeat: <u>Finding your "Get To Dos" is about giving yourself something. It's not about taking anything away</u>. For example, I can say to myself, "Every day, I shall have five servings of greens or whatever type of food is suggested to be super beneficial for me" or, "Before bed, I'll have an apple and an Isagenix fiber cookie!" You'll include your exercise plan also. For example: "I'm going to eat dinner, and then I'm going to walk to hear the outdoor concert (say it's twelve blocks away) and walk back (total of twenty-four blocks, which, when added to the ten blocks that I walked to and from the bank at lunchtime, puts me at thirty-four blocks), which puts me at four over my 30 block Q!" Yay!!!" You can find out what distance (miles, yards, whatever you choose to make your get-to-dos) streets, parks, etc. in your hometown equal.

There's another factor to consider. If you're reading this book, you're probably aware of the positive-thinking work that's been going on for a long while. Norman Vincent Peale's, *The Power of Positive Thinking* was published in 1945. Between the law of attraction and *The Secret*, we're all bombarded with the thought that if we put our minds to what we want, the universe will bring it to us. It sounds nice, but when I looked around, I met many people who were espousing the value of positive thoughts in one breath and telling me how rough their life was in the other! I was fortunate to meet, befriend, be coached by, and work with David Friedman. I mentioned David Friedman's theory before. Like me, he wondered why all of the positive thinkers weren't getting what they wanted in life. He added the idea that we don't do actions that will lead us to what we want because uncomfortable body sensations often come up when we think thoughts about getting what we want, and we'll do anything to avoid those sensations—and we usually don't even know we're doing that. *These uncomfortable sensations are often a result of somebody having told us we couldn't or shouldn't have what we said we wanted—or we were silly to think we could ever have that, given who we are. We often hear these negative statements about our possibilities when we're too young to properly evaluate what we're being told.*

This made me feel even stronger about my theory of getting rid of words that we were taught to negatively react to. David Friedman suggests we allow those uncomfortable sensations to be there and go after what we want anyway. The uncomfortable sensations can serve us. They usually mean we're heading toward what we want—because that's when they show up most. His book is listed in my unsolicited recommendations.

It's great if you can make up YOUR own TERM that doesn't put negative thoughts about getting into YOUR best shape into your mind.

The idea of developing a routine is ancient. Aristotle is known to have said, "We are what we repeatedly do. Excellence, then, is not an act but a habit."

The word "habit" has a more positive connotation than "routine." Books like *The 7 Habits of Highly Successful People* and others like it have helped lift the knee-jerk reaction to this word.

Your success is in your daily to-dos (give yours a name) and having them become as automatic as possible. Then, guess what? The results come without even worrying about it!

We Teach What We Needed to Learn

Another reason I'm writing this book is that I've discovered that the glamorous, well-built star I fantasized about and longed to be—in my grandma Fanny's attic in Bensonhurst, as I played alone for hours with my dolls and with the formal clothes my mom and grandma stored there—is, indeed, the glamorous star I am! I saw myself as the big, fat kid. That's why I was one. I did what a fat kid would do and ate what a fat kid would eat. In truth, I wasn't as fat as I thought I was, except for when I was ten and eleven years old and my self-esteem was dependent on being asked to dance at camp socials. I'm glad the practice of having such young children feel they need to attract a boyfriend or girlfriend isn't prevalent anymore.

The two places I felt truly comfortable were: 1. In my parents' living room alone in front of the TV. 2. Standing in front of people singing or acting or giving a talk. When I was on stage I was the "character" who was performing or giving the talk and not my dull, fat self. I even felt "less than" because I had a high IQ! Can you believe that? After WWII, when brilliant women were appreciated, the country seemed to feel we needed what I call over-the-top normalcy (the girls they called "dumb blondes" won the guys). The fashion of a particular time can be idiotic, and society can teach us some idiotic stuff! Guys have issues too. I'll bet some of you guys reading this book compared yourselves to the guys on the football team or whatever group was held in high esteem at your school or in your neighborhood. I remember when bald was automatically considered unattractive. Being born elsewhere can be a concern to many boys and girls. Having an accent from a foreign country or another state could pose problems (both imagined and learned).

In my early fifties, I studied and became a certified image consultant. During my training, I became fully aware of how gorgeous everyone is—I mean every person!

The reason someone may not come off gorgeous at first glance is that they just don't "get" they are. Some people unconsciously hide themselves in their clothing, often because they just don't know what harmonizes with them. I found that people who were very close to knowing what worked for them and who were in good—or at least fairly good—shape usually liked themselves. They were more likely to present themselves to the world in a manner that said, "I deserve to be here!" Would you believe that these people, the ones who need color and style training least, are almost always the first people who want to make appointments for color and style consultations? Believe it! Often, those who are in great need of help don't let themselves have it. It's possible they don't know they need help, but I feel they're burying that knowledge because it's painful and they think they'll have to work hard to look good. It would be like me saying I don't need an accountant! I can take care of it! Help!

In my early sixties, when my own body blew up and I started having pain, and cancer developed in me, I realized that clothes weren't the whole story. The vehicle we travel in and dress has to be vibrant and fit also.

My spiritual guide, Barbara Van Diest, dared to tell me I was looking older than I needed to. Bless her for giving me that feedback! I didn't really listen much for about two years. By the time I went on a one-on-one retreat with her in 2002, I'd blossomed into a lovely 163-pound creation! My neck was sagging, my arms were hanging, there were lines under my eyes, and I wasn't my previous bikini shape, to say the least! When I was with my son, he would help me down the subway stairs because my knees were in such pain. When I was alone, I clung to the railing and walked slowly. Everything hurt. My index fingers had bumps on the bones from osteoarthritis. My mom had those bumps when she got older. Barbara mentioned that she didn't think I needed to look that old or hurt that much. I'd spent my whole life conscious of my looks, if not my health. When Barbara saw I wasn't handling the issue myself, thankfully she stepped in.

There were previous times in my life when I'd gone through plans for dropping pounds and being fit. This time I realized I'd come up with something of my very own—and it was healthy, and it was working! Some of the products and nutritional findings weren't original. However, I had a way of wording how I was going about it that wasn't quite like anything I'd heard before. Barbara was floored with the way I was able to follow the healthy slimming "routine" (pardon the expression) and then maintain it. Please understand that I was, in part, using other people's systems—but not just one person's system—and while I was using the other systems, I was playing with them so they suited my style. *I made the systems I took from others my own. That's why I stuck with them.*

Gung ho!

As I succeeded, I felt better and better about myself. As my self-esteem grew, so did my ability to shed the extra weight and sagginess.

To repeat: I learned that in addition to the styles and colors we choose, how "in shape" we are gives a clue toward how we feel about ourselves. (I don't mean "model skinny" or "weight-lifter bulked up". I mean a healthy shape.)

In practicing image consulting, I find that people who love themselves are people who feel they deserve to have all the knowledge they can get about choosing a way of dressing that reflects who they are. I also find that people who truly love themselves are more likely to feel they deserve to be fit and, as I said, are usually the first to sign up for my "Be Fit & Fabulous From Fifty Forward" seminars. (Which I used to call "Find Your mini-Qs" seminars.

I'm Gung ho (remember the term "Gung ho"?) Gung ho means, truly committed and excited—to prove to you that you are a beautiful winner. As I said, it's my responsibility to do everything I can to give you more reason to love yourself. You're truly a winner right now! When you know that you are, you'll do what winner _____ would do.

(your name)

If you bought this book or received it as a gift or as part of a course you're taking, I know you care enough about yourself, or someone else cares about you, and you are, indeed, ready to walk this path. When you try it, and it works for you, you'll not only have a winner buried deep in your soul, but you'll feel and look and act like the winner you are!

PART II
Let the Games Begin

You Get to Design Your Own
"Whatever You Decide To Call
Your "Get-To-Dos"

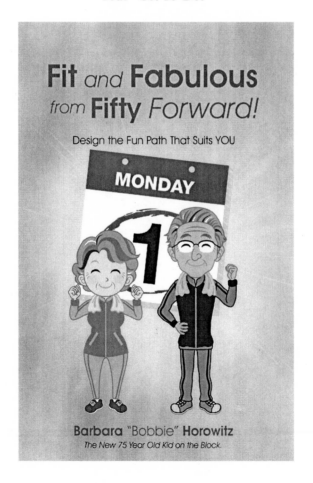

CHAPTER 6

Letting Go of Stress and Forgiving Yourself for Not Being as Fit as You Could Be

I've discovered that when beginning the process of getting your shape and health to be in the best condition they can be, it is helpful to forgive yourself for allowing (whether knowingly or not) yourself to be in less than great condition. How you talk to yourself holds an important key to your success in this (and probably any) area of your life.

Here's another thought that I find very helpful to keep in mind when thinking about my fitness: *what I am experiencing at this moment is the result of choices and decisions made in the past; what I will experience in the future depends on choices and decisions I make now.*

Happiness Is a Daily Decision

I emphasize the *daily*. Think of it as just being so for today. Don't worry about tomorrow. Write down your daily minimum "get-to-dos" now and then take each day as it comes.

To repeat: most modern-day philosophers are concluding that the results in our lives are a reflection of the thoughts we're holding. But how do those thoughts get there? Do we always plan which thoughts go into our heads at any time? We've been taught to think a lot of them. I hold that it's good to talk to ourselves and question our thoughts as though we are helping a friend we love. It can be easier to see a friend's foibles than our own.

Since I wrote my original book on this topic, *"Find Your mini-Qs (?) Reveal The Slim, Strong, Sexy Star You Truly Are at Age 50, 60, 70 and Beyond,"* I've started doing tapping, which is a method of stress reduction, almost every day. (More about that in chapter 15.)

Some would say that I'm being rash when I contend that if we spoke to others the way we've at times silently spoken to ourselves, we could be put in prison for some of the things we've said. I know *I* could. Sound crazy? I suggest you remind yourself to pay attention to what you say to yourself every day. I bet you come up with a threat to yourself every once in a while. You're a smart reader, so I think I can let this go now and feel confident that you get what I'm talking about.

Can we change our subconscious thoughts (our silent words) about our bodies? The answer is YES! We do have to allow for the old thoughts to slip in every once in a while - until they don't.

The most important thing I can think of that made it possible for me to stay at my optimum weight for almost 15 years now is that I've finally begun to be kinder to myself. In the past, I didn't realize how unkind I was being to me. Every once in a while, I still get angry with myself, but I do catch myself more quickly now. Instead of beating myself up, I think of my poor little cells crying, "Mommy, Mommy, we just wanted to you be happy!" If you learn nothing else, you'll be ahead of the game when you're kind to yourself. Being kind to yourself is certainly most important while you're designing and following your path to your optimum weight and fitness. Am I repeating myself? For most people, it takes repeating and repeating and repeating in different ways. Many people say they're kind to themselves, but when push comes to shove, I get that they chastise themselves when they don't follow through with their assignments. As with any "Aha!" you may get it, and then you may have to hear it again later to incorporate that "Aha!" into your daily life.

Tip: humor helps (I'll say it again!).

I've found something that helps me change my negative thoughts and talk to myself kindly. I've made up a playful, sad tone of voice that works for me. You can make up your own way of kindly playing with yourself. I say "Bobbie, Bobbie, (or like I wrote above, I also like "Mommy, Mommy") that was a negative thought. Please don't hurt my Bobbie!"

This sounds funny to me and gets me laughing.

Find things that make you giggle. Humor helps! Then I say to myself, "Hmmm, let's see where that (whatever the negative thought was) came from!" If I can think of it quickly (e.g., my mother said, "Don't fall! Don't be a klutz!" every time I left the house), I'll change it. However, in my heart I'm thinking (saying), *Oh sure! Right! I'm a thin, beautiful, successful, sought-after woman! Yeah, right!*

Then - once again, I need to get to forgive myself and try again. Here's where I use two different methods:

1. David Friedman's *The Thought Exchange*
2. Tapping (I especially recommend Nick Ortner's webinars, talks, and his book, *The Tapping Solution*.)

Both *The Thought Exchange* principles and tapping (or EFT as it is sometimes referred to) are helping me silence my critical voice that makes me nervous about who I am. I'm finally beginning to truly accept myself. I find that tapping for a few minutes every day keeps me from falling backward into unconsciously doubting myself as a worthy teacher, writer, performer, or producer.

In chapter 16, you'll find a link to Nick Ortner's website. You can read a chapter of *The Thought Exchange* at any time. If you're near NYC or Norwalk, Connecticut, you can work privately or in class with David Friedman.

In the past, when I thought the thought *"I'm a slender, beautiful, successful, sought-after woman"*, I'd feel a tightness in my solar plexus and find myself going to the refrigerator for a nosh. That tightness was an uncomfortable sensation that came on as a body memory of the past. "Bobbie is sweet. She's brilliant—but—her mind can be up there in the clouds sometimes." And when I was a teen, "She's a little heavy but a good student and nice." Or, "She's too dramatic." My sister Susie always "had her feet on the ground." I was the "artiste." Of course, if I were more theatrical or thinner than my mother, my family might have thought I wasn't what a daughter should be.

I was told that being "dramatic" or too concerned with fashion and not just looking clean and well bred was not what men were looking for. BUT - My dad loved fashion – and I'd read that fashion was about being well bred - so none of this made any sense!

My mom kept giving me the message that plain was better than dramatically gorgeous.

A lot of what our brains retain isn't necessarily logical. To repeat, we're usually not aware that what our brain is retaining is what was put into it when we were kids.

Another element to consider while designing your daily Get-To-Dos is: <u>forgiving yourself</u>. Know that you may have to hear this a few hundred times before you embrace it. I'm not being facetious. You may need several repetitions. Forgive yourself if, at any time, you don't follow what you've set for yourself. *When you can learn to forgive yourself for anything you do that isn't up to your standards, you'll be well on your way to attaining your goals.*

Note: Forgiving yourself doesn't mean that you stop believing you can and will do your daily "Get-To-Dos" every day. It sometimes takes having some fun with them and redesigning them or discovering ways to "fix" them in our memories. Know that you'll get there, and your "whatever you named them" (As you know, I call them mini-Qs) will start to engrave themselves in your brain. You'll naturally realize that doing your daily, weekly, and monthly get-to-dos is something you want to do because they work and nobody else gets to dictate your life!

You need to accept yourself as being perfect while you're the person you appear to be right now, in terms of how you're accomplishing your goals. *It's a learning process. It may take you a while to get the hang of just plowing into your daily get-to-dos as you live your day.* I might say I'm going to walk thirty blocks every day or a mile and a half every day, but it might take me a while to figure out how many blocks or miles there actually are between the beginning and end of my frequently travelled routes. I may have to allow myself to say, "Whoops! I didn't mean to park in front of the grocery. I meant to park on the top of the hill and walk down from there." There is no universal perfect. Give yourself a break and hug yourself with your thoughts—and then direct your thoughts to discovering some clue that will automatically (or almost automatically) get you to remember to park on top of the hill. It's not rocket science, but there are thinking patterns to develop. I bet that after a certain number of times of thinking about what trips in your life can be made by walking, you won't even need to think about it anymore.

Where you live can make a difference in terms of how simple it will be to plan exercise activities. So forgive yourself if it takes a week or so to have your movement Get-To-Dos in place.

Remember all those people's voices you were thinking about when we were discussing the choices you make? How many of those choices may not have come from your spirit but rather from an outside source? From someone or some group who taught you what they thought was the right way for everyone to be?

It's great to take a piece of paper each morning and write down the name of any person who comes to your mind who you think you might need to forgive for something and put the paper into "Forgiveness Folder" that you keep filed. It can be for the long-ago offense of someone telling you to "mouth" the song and not sing it in your school assembly or your mom yelling at you for not finishing your food. It can be for something that just happened, like your colleague speaking at a company meeting and forgetting to give you credit for helping him or her with work at a company meeting. The most important forgiveness work is forgiving yourself for not being what you would deem "perfect."

CHAPTER 7

Ask Yourself Questions

What Is My Lifestyle? How Can I Use It to Get Fit?

When and Where Do I Like to Eat? When Can I Walk &
What Can I Walk To and/or From a Place I Need To Be?
(Note: "O Blood Types" May Want To Put <u>Run</u> In Place of
Walk.) When Can I Lift Things in a Healthy Way? Etc.

Here we are at last! We're ready to look at your life and design a series
of daily "want-to-dos" that are geared to your lifestyle and health
needs. What I call the mini-Qs include the food, or type of food, you
choose to make part of your day and the number of times you choose
to eat a certain type of food each day, week, etc. For example: every
morning, I eat a protein that goes well with my body. I've matched
my food intake to my body needs, and you'll match your needs to
yours. They also include activities you engage in.

Note: I'll tell you what I found out goes well with my
body in chapter 11. I'll also make a few suggestions for
ways you can find out what goes well with your body.

Ask Yourself, "What's My Usual Day Like?"

This is not a test. The lists that follow are merely here to help you see how elements of your life have triggered you to eat at times other than your mealtimes or, perhaps, to choose foods you've chosen to please others, and then these choices became habitual. I used to crave sweets all the time. It was like muscle memory. My body thought that's what it needed. I can hear my wonderful Grandpa David laughingly saying things like, "Save up some room for dessert!" If the group says, "Let's order and share the large extra-cheese and fried-sausage pizza," do you have to go along? You're probably saying, "But I love the extra-cheese and fried-sausage pizza!" In the second part of this chapter, you'll learn how to choose foods that your body really likes – and, in time you'll get to crave those foods.

You'll see many pages with guidelines for lists you can make for yourself. These lists will help you fit your (I call them) "Get To Do's" into your daily lifestyle. Note: *I'm gifting you with the ability to download as many copies of these pages as you wish, once yiou've bought the book—at no charge. You'll be able to revise your lists as many times as you want to.*

Go to www.bobbiehorowitz.com and click on "Author." You'll see a spot for Page Lists. You'll be asked to make up a password, and you'll see instructions for downloading the pages you can write on.

It's best if you *quickly* fill in the blanks on the following lists— or see them in your mind if that works better for you. Note that the physical act of writing things down helps most people retain information.

While you already know this stuff, it can be a great help to break it down to see where and when your eating choices may be distorted by other people's wishes and by other obligations you have.

First, let's take a look at your household. You can choose:

- I live alone.
- I live with my wife/husband.

- My child (children) lives with me.
- My grandchildren live with me.
- Roommates live with me.
- I live in a senior residence with many people.
- I have live-in help.
- I have daily help that comes in.
- I have a health aide that comes in twice a week.
- *Anything else that describes your situation.*

Now let's take a look at your usual day's clock. Fill in the times for each activity. If you think of other situations that exist in your household or your schedule, add them in.

- I wake up at _____.
- I eat breakfast at home.
- I usually eat breakfast out at _____ (time).
- I usually eat breakfast out at _____ (place).
- I leave for work at. _____.
- I leave for my friend's house (my club, class, etc.) at _____.
- I have a health aide come in at. _____ o'clock.
- A physical trainer comes in _____ days/week at _____ (time).
- I take my work breaks at _____ (time/s).

> Note: I now work from home, and I find that it's still good to set up these plans. When I set up plans, I tend to get more work done and have more personal time. It's easy to lose personal time when you work from home.

At the beginning of a new set of plans to accomplish something, I find that when I set my plan up as though it was new each day (even if it is the same as the day before), it feels less like the same old routine. I suggest you try this. When I was restoring my fitness, once I was truly into the daily plan, I just went on with it each morning.

For everyone I've worked with, after a few days, rewriting the same plan became unnecessary. It became like brushing their teeth.

Put down your recurring weekly and monthly activities as well. For example: Tuesday night is my weekly singing class, and the first Monday of each month, I have my book club meeting.

I'll also set up my personal and household chore breaks each day.

I'll also list the time for each day's chores, including household chores. I list the time in case I'm relying on a doctor's or another company's schedule to get things completed during my day.

For example:

- I usually eat lunch at home at ____ o'clock.
- I usually eat lunch out at_____o'clock (time).
- I usually eat lunch out at (place).
- I close shop at home at _____ o'clock.
- I close shop at the office at.____ o'clock (if you have an office).
- I usually meet people after work at.____ o'clock.
- I come home from work at.____ o'clock.
- I eat dinner at home at _____ o'clock.
- I usually eat dinner out at _____o'clock
- I usually eat dinner out at _____(place).

Feel free to add other possibilities so the list reflects your day.

Weekly and Monthly Obligations

- I'm usually out on this day of the week at _____ (time) for _____ (name of event).

I'll make the form shorter now. I think you've gotten the idea:

I go to meetings, and I bring my dinner with me.. bring a snack and eat when I get home, or the event provides the food.

Next, list your household responsibilities, if any… if you have more than a dozen of these responsibilities, just list the number you have. Include the time you usually do the tasks.

1. Example: (Task) @ (8:00 a.m.)
2.
3.
4.
5.
6.
7.
8.
9.
10.

CHAPTER 8

Your Body's History Dealing with Different Foods—Questions, Questions, and More Questions

It's good to keep asking questions while you're designing your path. It's great for you to know as much about your life—as it is now—as you can. This will help you make our "eating day" feel like it's yours rather than a day that's been imposed on you. You get to focus on *your* physicality (what your body composition is) and also, to a large degree, the things you were taught (both helpful and not helpful) when you were young.

It's good to make a list of as many things as you can think of about your vehicle (i.e., your body). Wouldn't you want to know as much as you could about a car your owned?

These are some questions you should get answers for if you don't already know the answers:

- Find out which foods are best for your body type and blood type. Take into consideration any injuries, diseases you've caught, etc. and may have had in your life.

- For body type, you may want to consult a licensed physical trainer as well as a physician. Well informed trainers should have learned very specific things about how a particular body type works and what feeds it well.

- To find out the foods that are best for you, those you should avoid, and those that are neutral for your system, ask your physician and also ask a nutritionist. If your doctor and the nutritionist disagree with each other, I suggest getting a third opinion. Many licensed physical trainers have had education in nutrition also. They should know that different blood types do best with exercises that fit their needs. We're not all the same.

While this can sound time-consuming, it will save you lots of time once you get started, and I bet you'll get great results. I'm going to give an example of a project that's much more difficult and uncertain than you getting into the best shape possible and maintaining it. However, I think you get the idea of why - <u>asking questions before you start is important.</u>

Think of a Broadway producer deciding the best way to put up a new musical show. There are many aspects to each show, and as a producer, the more questions you ask (and get the best possible answers for) before you plan your budget, raise the money, choose and rent your theater, cast your actors, and hire your staff, the more chance you have of succeeding. The producer (or team of producers) will most likely have put up a couple of out-of-town small-theater tryouts before putting the musical up on Broadway.

Think of getting in shape like producing a show. Your job is much easier than the producer's job is. You can also have fun with it. Know that you're letting your work of art shine through to the world, just as the musical's producer is inspired to present a work of art to the world!

One thing you can know is that your work of art is an excellent one.

Once again, note that you can keep revising your plan as you see things work or not work. That said, *the more questions you've gotten answered by pros, before you start, the simpler your path will be.*

Note: Back in the thirties, forties, fifties, and sixties, many parents made their children eat things that really didn't agree with them. The parents didn't know they were doing this. If they did, I'm sure they wouldn't have cajoled their children to eat or drink things our particular bodies wouldn't digest well. They were taught that kids had to have these foods.

Oh that orange juice!

I remember that when I was in kindergarten (and it probably also occurred before that), my mother wouldn't allow me to leave in the morning without having my orange juice. I recommend you become familiar with Dr. Peter D'Adamo's books about blood types. While you needn't obsess about it, I suggest you find out your blood type. It's very easy to do. Your doctor probably has it in his/her records. I have blood type A. I learned that A's have more trouble dealing with acid than O blood types do. My poor stomach was on fire for most of the morning after that orange juice! I wanted ice cream all the time because that seemed to soothe it. Of course, I wasn't allowed to have ice cream in the morning. Now I know that dairy isn't the best thing for me, but some dairy products are neutral for me. Now if I crave that smooth sweetness, I'll get frozen yogurt. It may not be my most beneficial food, but it's neutral and not harmful. I don't crave soothing ice cream all the time. In fact, I just realized that I hardly ever think about ice cream anymore, unless I'm in a restaurant and would like something smooth and cool like frozen yogurt and they don't have it on the menu. I'll wait till I get home to have a spoonful of frozen Tofutti or Yogurt. I really craved ice cream as a child because the acid in the orange juice and other foods I was fed was irritating my stomach lining, and the ice cream felt soothing.

We've also learned a lot about cholesterol since I was young. When I first heard cholesterol being talked about, all fat was assumed problematic. Now we know there is a form of fatty acid we need that actually helps control our cholesterol. There are supplements like omega fatty acid capsules to help us be sure to have it in our bodies. I used to have very high cholesterol, and now I'm in the low-normal range! I'm thankful that my doctor knew about and favored a natural means of healing. I'll mention this and other products from various companies that I've found to be excellent in chapter 11.

Paying attention to your body will help you make choices that turn out to be fun for you!

Note: I stopped eating oranges, tomatoes, and peppers about eleven years ago. Since choosing not to eat these foods, I don't have stomach pains, and I even find myself forgetting to keep antacids in my home in case anyone who comes over needs one! I've not needed even one antacid or "tummy pill" since I learned which foods can cause me problems and which benefit me!

<u>I can't say I gave up these foods because</u> after a year or so, (You'll probably need to give yourself sometime to get over your hankerings – but, I bet you'll be surprised at the results.) I never thought about wanting them again. <u>I really didn't give up anything.</u> <u>I received a lot by feeling better.</u>

Next we'll look at a few lists that you can make. They're good to keep near your fridge. You'll probably have even more than fifty foods on each of your lists. I've written out a few lines to give you an idea of how to proceed. Add your extras to your list. If you have fewer, leave the additional lines blank. In time, you may find you have more beneficial foods than you thought. Feel free to add more than fifty foods or list fewer if that's the case for you, and revise the list as you learn more about food and your body. You can write them on the Food List page. I like to number the foods to make them easier to see quickly. Tape the page to the inside of your kitchen cabinet door.

Be sure to include a section each for meat (unless meat is not good for you), poultry, fish, vegetables, grains, dairy, nuts, seeds, oils, beans, fruits, spices, coffee and teas, and supplements. You can write it by hand on paper. It can help to have it on your computer, in case something happens to the paper copies; but it's not necessary.

Foods That Are Beneficial for Me

Meat

(You may or may not have meat on your list. If meat is a food you should avoid, don't have the category on your list. Since my blood type is "A positive", I don't have meat on mine. It's not that a little will kill me, but the acid in meat can cause damage to my system—and it did—over time. It's great to feel healthy now! Others, especially people with blood type O need meat and its acidity.)

1. _____
2. _____
3. _____
4. _____
5. _____
6. _____
7. _____
8. _____
9. _____
10. _____

Poultry

1. _____
2. _____
3. _____
4. _____
5. _____
6. _____

7. _____

8. _____

9. _____

10. _____

Make sections for vegetables, fruits, grains, dairy products, etc.

Foods I Can Label as Neutral for Me (This will refer to YOU)

They won't benefit you to any great degree, but they're okay for you to eat. You'll probably have more foods in this category. Again, divide your list into food categories, including meat, poultry, fish, vegetables, grains, dairy, nuts, seeds, oils, grains, beans, fruits, spices, coffee and teas, supplements, etc.

Foods I Should Avoid (Meaning YOU should avoid)

Note that I don't generally keep foods that I should avoid in my home. I sometimes will buy something from this list if company is coming and I know they'd want that particular food. It might be beneficial for them.

> Note: If you live with someone or are in a relationship with someone you see often, if these foods are beneficial for him/her, I would think you'd want to keep them on hand for that person. While this could potentially lead to arguments, if you're clear about it upfront, the two of you can create a fun game out of it! Plus, you can both feel better because you're eating foods that are good for you, respectively.

Again, I put the number of foods in randomly; create as many lines as you need for each list.

49

CHAPTER 9

Your Daily (the Name You Gave Your Daily Get-to-Dos) for What to Eat When

Remember: you deserve to be the star you truly are!

Note: As you know, I call these my "mini-Qs." You probably have your own name for them by now.

It Helps to Begin Each Day with Gratitude

Before you get out of bed, say, "Thank you!" Thank yourself and your home and your food and life!

It adds fun to know your dominant style of look. It can help put fun into the start of your day. Your personality style usually (but not always) follows the style of your look. I'll talk more about how you can find out about your personal style in chapter 12.

If your main style is dramatic like mine, you may want to strike a film star wake-up pose. If you're a "Dramatic Style Guy", think of yourself in a silk robe, and if you're a dramatic female, imagine yourself in a silk or velvet robe with a fur (okay, faux fur) collar. Sit up in bed with your legs over the side, stretch your toes down toward the floor, and stretch your arms high to the ceiling. Let your arms lower and arch your back and sensually roll your shoulders. If your physicality doesn't allow for this, then do what you can to get an "ummmm" good feeling. Delicious! Breathe in and smile a big feeling-good smile and breathe out with an audible, pleasurable "Mmmmmm!" and say, "Thank you!" softly to yourself.

Reverend Carlos Anderson, a Unity minister, has a wonderful way to get the day going. After your "Thank You" (which was my method) he suggests your going to the window, looking outside and saying "This is the best day ever!!" I think he's on to something!

Note that like me, your main style may not be the style of your dominant coloring. It is the same for many (most) people; but not for everyone (not for me). My coloring is natural while my style is dramatic. I hope I'm enticing you to find out more about your color and style. It will greatly help you bring out the star you are.

Contact me on my site and I'll let you know when I'm giving a webinar. (I plan to restore the webinars I held now that I've had cataracts removed from both eyes and can once again fully see color!)

My Image Consulting site is www.bobbiehorowitz.com. Look at my schedule for upcoming workshops.

If you're dominant style is natural, you can fluff out your thick hair with your hand, make a fist, push it up toward the ceiling, and say, "Thank you for this brand-new day!"

If you're major style is gamin, or what some call pixyish, clap your hands, bounce up and down on your bed, and giggle as you say, "Thank you!"

If you're a mainly classic style, sit up like a gentleman or lady and softly clasp your hands (or put them in prayer position, if that pleases you) and say, "Thank you!"

Some of us are clearly one style, but most people are a combination of styles. Most of us have a dominant style and then sub-styles. If you don't yet know style is, until you do, try them all and say: "Thank you!" with each.

Note: <u>In chapter 11, you'll find out how to get in touch with me for a color/style analysis.</u> If you live far from New York and can't get here, I'll recommend someone near to where you live. Again, I hope I've enticed you to do this. It made a big difference in my life.

Whatever your spiritual beliefs are or even if you have none, I've discovered that "Thank you!" seems to mitigate many of the angry thoughts that might pop up in the morning. You don't want to fight the thoughts because that will just make them stronger. I've learned that anger sometimes pops up in the <u>morning</u>. I checked out my theory that I wasn't the only one to experience this by Googling the topic. I was amazed by the number of articles I found on the subject of "anger in the morning". There were over 85 million listings! I find that saying the morning "Thank you" and then also saying, "You must be here to teach me something about myself. Thank you," should any negative thought come into my mind during the day, seems to make the negative thought less real and make it easier to laugh at.

Look at the list you made of what your day is like. You've gotten your checkup, and you know what supplements will help you and which, if any, may be harmful. Plan to repeat what you put down for the next couple of weeks. Then check it out again and keep what's working and modify or ditch what's not.

Helpful hint about noshing (Yiddish for grabbing food when it's not mealtime): After dinner is often the time I want to "go at it" - in terms of eating. I know that about myself. I find it a big help to make the same choice every night. Choosing the same thing every night as a treat (i.e., make it an "I get to have!") makes it more fun for me, and therefore, I'm much more likely to keep it light and make it a habit. (I know "habit" is a dirty word, but it's what works)

The whole Q concept is to make it easy to develop good habits—without thinking of them as dull routines all the time.

Also, remember that going to the fridge for cake and ice cream every night is a habit.

What time of day do you find yourself most wanting to nosh?

Your kitchen is now filled with the foods you like and that are healthy for you to eat. When you wake up in the morning, you haven't eaten for several hours, so be sure to choose some protein and some greens for alertness. It's also great if it's easy to prepare. Oh, did I say that it doesn't have to be what's become known as a breakfast food? It doesn't.

Supplements

Be sure you have the morning, afternoon, and nighttime supplements that your homeopathic doctor and/or nutritionist said were beneficial for you. If you don't have this information yet, you can find out more in chapter 16, where I give you my unsolicited recommendations. Also, take any medication that has been prescribed for you.

Note: I like to get second opinions regarding supplements and especially for prescribed medicines—just to be sure. I showed the Isagenix and MAX supplements I use to my doctor, who agreed that they're working for me. They worked so well for me that I no longer take any prescription drugs. I certainly would take a prescription medicine for a short while if two doctors I trust agreed that it would be important for me to take it.

Take supplements in the order your doctor told you to. My general practitioner agreed that the supplements I was taking seemed to have done a great deal of good for me, based on my past conditions. He also agreed with the sequence in which I took them.

Some are taken before meals, some with meals, etc. Most are helped by clean water.

Questions have recently been brought up concerning amounts of water to drink. We don't have final answers yet. Perhaps gulping liquid, including water, may not be the best thing for many people. Drinking throughout the day feels right to me. I've recently heard that a glass of water before bedtime is healthy, and it seems fine thus far. I don't claim to be an expert on sleep patterns. I have no trouble sleeping.

When I was a kid, we never drank water in our house. We drank Coca Cola and sometimes Seltzer. I'm thankful I survived. My parents didn't know that it wasn't the best. Almost everyone living in today's environment on earth (wide-open spaces not excluded) needs some supplement and some way to cleanse the system of the toxins that are in our air, water, earth, and food. "Toxin" is a very popular word now, and there's a good reason for it. We've made a lot of technological progress and - in doing so - we've dirtied up the planet. I have a feeling that in a few hundred years or so, the human body will adapt to better handle toxins. We've adapted to many things as conditions on our planet have changed. I believe that's why the different blood types developed.

I do use a water filter on my faucets and pour the water into glass containers and put drops of an alkaline PH Booster in the water.

I've probably overestimated the number of supplements you take on the following list. Just fill in the ones you *get* to take.

Tip: For the times of day you're out (e.g., for afternoon and/or evening supplements), it's great to take one envelope for the group of supplements you take for each time of day and put those envelopes into one slightly larger envelope. Plastic bags might be easier, but I try to avoid plastic when possible. If you use plastic, you can first wrap a tissue around them. You can always keep the bags filled. This way, if you get a last-minute call to go out, you don't have to think about it. Use a magic marker to write the time to take each set of supplements on the envelope for that time (e.g., a.m., p.m., anytime, dinner, etc.). You'll probably get to know your list fairly quickly. It helps to have the lists so that when changes need to be made, you just take off the old and add the new until you get used to it and know them without having to think about them.

My morning (if any) supplements are:

a.

b.

c.

My lunchtime (if any) supplements are:

a.

b.

c.

My evening (if any) supplements are:

a.

b.

c.

My bedtime (if any) supplements are:

a.

b.

c.

My Breakfast-at-Home Possibilities Are …

Note that you can list combinations of things if you wish. For example: I find it easier to eat basically the same thing for breakfast every day. I know this particular breakfast gives me what I need, and I've grown to love it. I play around with it to make it slightly different on different days. I'll give you my recipes in the final section of this book. If you prefer to vary your breakfast on different days, you can list a group of things to choose from.

> For example: an *egg* + *half a piece of rye toast with a small amount of ricotta* + *a cup of chopped broccoli* + *one cup of organic coffee with a teaspoon of cream* or – *one small bowl of Amaranth flakes* + *half a cup of soymilk (depending on your dairy tolerance)* + *a peach (organic is always good)* + *one cup of green tea.*

You can choose from any of the foods that benefit you in their portions for any breakfast. Pretty soon, you won't need to measure foods. You'll just know how much of each thing to use. That's what Aristotle meant by "habit." Habits are good things—if they're good habits! They're the way we get things accomplished. My goal is to make the whole habit issue a non-issue.

If coffee is beneficial for you, then you can add a cup of coffee or you can add tea. Some people are better with green tea than black tea. A soft drink doesn't include sodas for almost everyone. Some people can handle carbonation, and others are better off without it. You can also add some of the foods that are neutral for you.

My Breakfast-Out Possibilities Are …

List the dishes that are beneficial for you that you're pretty sure you'll find in the diners or restaurants you'd usually go to for breakfast. This can often prove a challenge. It's great to carry the lists of foods that are beneficial, neutral, and not good for you when you go out until you really know them by heart. Every once in a while, you'll be in a restaurant that has a menu with few choices for you. Try to find a choice that has mostly beneficial ingredients for you, and feel free to tell your waitperson that you wish to leave out

<u>the ingredients that aren't beneficial</u>. You can explain why if you're asked. Most waiters and waitresses will try to accommodate you. However, if, for example, you ask about leaving tomatoes out of a salad, and the salad is already chopped up, you may not be able to have them remove the tomatoes. I'm fanatic about following my list, but unless you're highly allergic to a food, a few strips of a tomato won't kill you. However, try not to eat the unbeneficial foods too often.

List your eating times for the rest of your day.

My at-Home Midmorning Snack Possibilities Are …

- My Lunch-at-Home Possibilities Are …
- My Lunch-Out Possibilities Are …
- My at-Home Afternoon Snack Possibilities Are …
- My Afternoon Snack Possibilities Out Are …
- My at-Home Dinner Possibilities Are …
- My Dinner-Out possibilities Are …
- My Before-Bedtime Snack Possibilities Are …

(I always have these at home, and I keep this list short. I have only one or two choices. You could add a few more if you wish.)

CHAPTER 10

Your Life Is Your Gym

Design your get-to-dos (whatever you've named yours) for strength and tone.

Note: remember to ask questions.

Just as you asked your doctors and researched the foods that would be best for your body, ask questions of your orthopedist, internist, and any other doctors you see if they have suggestions for you. Of course ask your physical trainer, if you have one, and get second opinions.

Not everyone's body is the same. Your body may need to jump and run - or slow long-distance walking and slow bending and stretching may be what your body reacts to best. One person's body may do best with lifting medium weights up and down quickly while another person's body may react best to lifting heavy weights for just a few lifts and very slowly. I was amazed at how well I did lifting weights that were so heavy I'd never believed I could lift them! As I built strength, I used 130-pound weights that I lifted and brought down to a slow count of thirty, and I did only three lifts. It took me a while to be able to lift that weight. I built up to it. Find a trainer who's up on the latest research. Once you're sure of what's right for you in the different movement areas, you can work with a trainer once in a while just to keep things in check.

If you see a series of classes you think are right for you, it's best to get them to allow you to try it out for one or two sessions to make sure it is right for you—or at least pay for only one or two sessions. This way, if the movements used in the class aren't right for your body, you won't have to pay for the whole series.

I repeat, yet again, that you can revise until you find what works for you.

Here we go!

- "Up in the morning, out on the job," from "That Lucky Ole Sun," lyrics by Haven Gillespie
- "Tote that barge and lift that bail," from "Ole Man River," (once again) lyrics by Oscar Hammerstein

Remember the lines from these old songs?

Think of life a few millennia ago. That's not really such a long time in the grand scheme of things. Even just a few hundred years ago or less, homeowners had to pump water from the well. They'd climb up a hill and pick veggies. They had to carry chamber pots and wash clothes by hand in the river. Their bodies expected to have to do more physical work than most of today's life gives us. Today, some people actually engage in rigorous physical activity on the job, but most of us don't. Even today's farmers have more machinery to help them than farmers had a couple of centuries ago. It's no wonder that our bodies have become less taut from the daily grind. Our daily grind in the twenty-first century is probably more mental than physical.

Interestingly, throughout history, there have been people who were waited on and didn't have to work a lot. Cleopatra is reputed to have been humongous around the middle. That was desirable then. It meant you were well-to-do. It was thought to make it easier to carry a fetus. Wide-hipped women were worth more camels. I learned this from a sheik in a camp of nomads when I visited Israel in 1962.

My treasured life coach, the late Barbara Van Diest, got me to see that it's beneficial to go out and take a walk before doing anything else. (For the ladies: If you wish to, it's fine to take a moment to put on a little lipstick and eyeliner if you live in a town or in the city where you'll see people and it will make you feel more vital and alive. Women are still wearing makeup, and until that practice ends (which it may never), it can lift up your spirit.) This outing makes you part of the world and can give you energy. You can count it as part of your daily exercise movements, and it gets you in contact with life.

If you're already committed to a training regime in a gym or at home with a trainer and it's working for you, I say stick with it. If you belong to a health club, have taken advantage of your membership, have enjoyed going to it for a substantial amount of time, and have kept up a weekly schedule giving you the exercise you need, I say, "Bravo! Brava! You don't have to fix what's not broken."

I repeat that I would suggest asking your doctor about specific exercises your body may need or any that may not be best for your body.

By the way, I learned that different exercises are beneficial for the different blood types. It sounded crazy to me, but when I visited Dr. D'Adamo, I learned why, and it's made a great difference for me. You'll find his information in chapter 16.

While it's important to move, I always say, "There just may be something I don't know. A question can't hurt." For example, if you have low bone density and you're working out by stretching and bending only, you may want to add weight-bearing exercises to your daily mini-Qs or add walking, which is a weight-bearing exercise. If your doctor isn't familiar with how exercise affects your body, ask to see a practitioner who has some expertise in this area.

Cautionary note: I put this cautionary note in because I learned that I needed to refrain from taking a Pilates class that used the machines designed for Pilates. I'd had foot surgery, and I learned that the way you grounded yourself with your feet on the machines could damage my feet as they are now. Is that a usual concern? No! However, there are cases in which you should opt out of using certain pieces of equipment or doing certain exercises. So, especially if you'd had surgery or an injury, check it out first.

If you like working out at your gym and you're happy with this method, then your to-dos will be the exercises and the repetitions of each. I hope you're aware that you're also getting exercise when you're engaged and active in life. Yay!

If you can't seem to get yourself to a gym consistently due to your busy schedule, take a look at your daily activities. Are there places in your day when you can sneak in exercise without taking a break for it? For example, can you *walk* to a store or an appointment?

Also, if you go to a gym or you're fortunate enough to have a gym in your building complex, you can always use the treadmill or a track if your building has one.

I think cities like New York make life easier for exercise. Maybe I think this because I live in Manhattan. I'm aware that I can get very chauvinistic at times!

I walk everywhere. It's always fun. Here's a sneak preview of one of my mini-Qs. One of my daily mini-Qs for exercise is walking a minimum of thirty blocks per day no matter what! Thirty blocks equals a mile and a half in Manhattan. I almost always exceed this daily mini-Q, but remember, it's my mini, not my maxi. I'm thinking of upping it since, for the past few days, I've been walking fifty or more blocks.

I sometimes break it up. I can shop for groceries and go to the bank in the morning. For me, that's sixteen blocks (or more than three-quarters of a mile) back and forth, and I don't even notice I've walked. That's just over half my mini-Q! I get a kick out of planning my day in a way that ensures I fit in lots of walking. I can easily walk three miles. I plot chores along the way—chores that might make the walk even longer than it would usually be. So it doesn't seem like I'm exercising—I'm just living my life!

Just because others aren't walking in the suburbs doesn't mean you can't! You can also garden in the suburbs. If you like to garden, do as much of it yourself as you can. Lifting the containers of plant food, etc. is good exercise, as is lifting the water containers. I love to garden and at one point I actually created a roof garden. If gardening isn't your thing and you don't play a sport (the suburbs are havens for golf courses and tennis clubs), there is always the shopping mall. Many malls are large, and walking around them can give you some distance. You can also shop for food, etc. at many of the malls, so you can get your daily chores done too. It's a good idea to park as far as you safely can from the store you need to go into on any given day.

Do you know what got me to decide to walk a minimum of thirty blocks a day? I started walking a lot when there was a NYC transit strike! I had an office then. I walked to work during the strike. It was fun! So I continued to walk after the strike was over. The distance to work from my apartment at the time was only half of my mini-Q today! Walking both ways would equal my mini-Q today. I'm ten years older now, and the length of that walk seems like nothing to me now!

Helpful hint: I find that I'm more able to get to the mini-Qs (get-to-dos) in my work life if I do at least some of my walking as early in the day as possible. Even if you have a great city or nature view from inside your home, if you physically can, there's something about getting out into the world that gets most people cooking. The participants in my workshops agreed that this helped them.

I recently realized that I haven't been getting outdoors as early as I had been. Being in the gym with people in the morning is good, and I still find it a help—to get my brain going—to go outside for an early walk, even it if it's just for a couple of blocks.

Do you have times during the day that you could fit in some isometrics and/or exercises? I've been doing isometrics and facial exercises at home for about six years. I do most of them before I even leave my bedroom in the morning. I usually do the last part of the facial exercises I've chosen while watching the morning weather report.

By isometrics, I mean things like clenching buttocks and pressing hands together.

One very bright fellow, a professor, in a summer seminar I held a few years ago found he could do isometric arm, stomach, and butt exercises at the bus stop while waiting for his bus. Waiting in line anywhere provides a great place to exercise. It's never too late to learn. I now clench my buttocks while seated on the bus. I'm the only person on the bus who hopes for traffic!

Again, you don't have to actually write these down. I do find writing things down to be helpful for absorbing them into my consciousness. It is important, however, to at least think of what different movements you can include and picture yourself doing a whole bunch of them.

Morning Exercise Movements I Can Do—and Where I Can Do Them

Note: There are many movements you can choose from. If you have paralysis or dysfunction in your limbs or other areas of your body, you'll have fewer choices. Remember, however, that this is about being *your* possible fittest. If you're in a wheelchair, you can work with that. Whatever your level of possible fitness may be, you probably won't choose to do all of them each day. They're actually part of your chores and activities, and many are done on a weekly or other basis. They're the things you do in life. You can add to the exercise elements in each activity when you think of them as exercise activities. For example, you can press you hands together when lifting your laundry out of the washing machine. You certainly may list additional movements to those I've listed.

Again, it's helpful to write a list of things you'll do—things like sweeping the floor, doing laundry, cleaning out file cabinets, etc. I work from home. I spend time at my computer writing and connecting with people and coaching. It helps me to get up from my computer and do actual exercise movements. These can look something like this:

9:30–10:00 a.m. Write book.

10:00–10:05 a.m. Stand and stretch my arms up to the ceiling. Hold that position for a count of ten and then slowly bend from the waist and reach my arms until my palms rest on the floor.

Continue writing your list for the morning. If you choose to bend and your arms can't touch the floor, make the bend go as far as your arms can reach down. Change the distances of the stretch as soon as you find you're comfortably able to reach the position you listed. You'll find yourself making progress in your ability to rest your palms flat on the floor when you bend from the waist. Then add to the number of times you stretch down till you reach about ten times.

On your next break, you can stretch your arms up toward the ceiling, or you can do both during one break, perhaps halving the number of times you do each.

You can do this after every half hour on the computer. If you haven't the time for this—and most of us truly do, if we stay focused— you can do your moves every forty-five minutes or whatever works for you. The idea is that your mind begins to incorporate the idea that your daily living is automatically filled with exercise.

Most people I've worked with have found they progress quite quickly in their ability to move different parts of their body, resulting simply from having followed a pattern of moving for a few days. I believe our bodies naturally want to be in the best shape they can be.

Not that many hundreds of years ago, someone in the household walked to the well or lake carrying a big pitcher to the water, then filled the pitcher and walked back, having to carry the heavy, liquid-filled pitcher! Exercise was part of life for the average person.

You can follow the same routine but use different movements for the remaining periods of time in each day.

You can include, for example, any of the following:

Afternoon Break Activities I Can Do —and Where I Can Do Them

Dinnertime Movements I Can Do—and Where I Can Do Them

Nighttime Movements I Can Do—and Where I Can Do Them

I think you get the picture.

I like to write my activities down in my date book. I use the monthly books from Franklin Planner, and I explain why in chapter 16. If you prefer, you could also put them on your Internet calendar. I find it helps to write EX (for exercise)—or something that represents exercise to you—next to it.

You'll be accomplishing two things at once. I think you'll find yourself moving with more concentration when your mind realizes you're getting exercise in your activities as well as accomplishing a chore or having fun. You'll also look at your work times and chore times in a slightly different way. I did. Now I want everything I choose to do to benefit my healthy lifestyle. (Well, I sometimes need to remind myself that I'm living to totally benefit myself. I've been finding help in this area and will discuss more in chapter 16.)

CHAPTER 11
How You Can Strike a Hit in Eight Possible "Strike-Out Situations"

Note that this chapter hasn't changed much from the chapter on this topic that's in my original book. Many people thanked me for writing it.

The eight situations are those in which you're dealing with other people. When we enter the realm of choosing the foods we'll eat when we go out with people, we enter a realm that's about our dealing with group psychology in addition to our own. Of course, it really does boil down to our own psychology because it's about how we choose for ourselves while we're in the group.

1. Travel

All of the situations in this section have travel as one of the components. Travel gives you another reason to set up another set of "mini-Qs"(your name for them) for yourself.

- I notice a psychological party-time/nervous-time feeling that I get when I travel— even if it's for business. Part of that is an apprehension of the unknown. Remember what I mentioned in chapter 2 about avoiding scary body sensations that come up when we think of actually going after what we want. Just let the scary feelings be there and go ahead with the choice you make anyway.

- If you are invited to a major cocktail event while on your trip, you needn't turn it down to keep your word to yourself. Just let your feelings be there. Those feelings will probably include cravings—unless you haven't eaten and those cravings are there because you really should eat something. Travel can be exciting. You can gain a wonderful lifetime memory—without gaining a pound! If I hadn't been willing to cross the pond to produce a musical in London, I would never have gotten to hug and befriend wonderful Princess Michael of Kent who was the guardian angel of the Jermyn Street Theatre. (Shhh, don't tell anyone! You're not supposed to touch royalty!) I also got to bow to Queen Elizabeth at an event that honored producer Cameron Mackintosh. (I had to name drop so you can see that this was truly thrilling for me!) I didn't yet have the mini-Q concept—but I'm glad, in any case, I went to the events. I would have followed my mini-Qs (had I known about them).

  - In truth, I was following my mini-Qs in the area of my work! I just hadn't named them mini-Qs yet. Doing mini-Qs (consistent daily activities) is what got the show produced. I wouldn't have been at those events had I not produced that show and met the wonderful people I met. Thank you again, "mini-Qs"! <u>NOTE: The term you make up for yourself - that deals with the minimum "get to dos" you need to do each day to accomplish your fitness goals - can be used for any project you wish to accomplish.</u>

- Ask yourself how any time changes that come with your trip may affect the health "Get To Dos" you set up for yourself. If there is a time change, be sure to pack a healthy snack (e.g., for breakfast if the hour is later than you're used to). When I travelled to London, I hadn't yet come up with the mini-Q idea, and I must say, my compatriot and I had at least four meals a day for the first few days we were there. I was starving the first morning or so due to the time difference. It was five hours later for me in London. The best way to deal with time differences when you travel is to prepare for them at home. Note and prepare for time changes. They can upset your inner hunger clock. I was still in my gaining weight stage. I was unconsciously doing my mini-Qs as a producer but not as a healthy eater. Once you have your "Get To Dos", you'll be fine if you follow them.

2. Holidays

Note: Cheer for holidays! Fun is a good thing! We can have fun *and* choose healthy foods and activities for ourselves!

- At the end of this chapter, you'll learn how to form your guilty list. *On a holiday, I advise you to allow yourself one small bite of one or two things you have.n your guilty list—if those things are linked with the holiday you're celebrating. You can join the crowd with one small bite.* Think of the meaning that particular food has when you take your one bite and savor the joy of partaking in the ritual. I don't even think of wanting a whole piece of birthday cake anymore. It's become my delight to have *a contributory bite.* This works especially well for your giving heart. You feel like you really made your contribution to the celebration by enjoying that *one bite.*

- *Most of our holidays are linked to a tradition of food.* Very often, they're the foods of the countries in which celebrations for that holiday started. Sometimes they're the foods that were popular at celebrations our ancestors experienced in their old country. Most of us were brought up linking holidays with eating. Halloween often starts an eating spree that continues until New Year's Day. If you ask people what Halloween is about, I'll bet that most will answer, "Halloween parties with ghosts and goblins and/or pumpkin pies." They may not know that the title of the evening is "All Hallows' Eve." I Googled "Halloween drinks" and got about 73,600 results! Many of these were nonalcoholic and sweet for the kids. Our holiday eating habits are developed at an early age.

- *Holidays often relate to memories of people having less than we (as a civilization) do and then being brought through lack to greater prosperity.* It's easy to understand that food is a big deal in that case. I think of Passover, which celebrates the Israelites' liberation from Egypt. They may have not all have been slaves, meaning totally unpaid servants, but they were certainly relegated to the servant class. They had to flee with the food they could carry. There was no food in the desert until manna was provided. Therefore, having food is giving thanks to God in this case.

- *On holidays, for many, the true focus of the holiday is a dinner.* In certain years, I experience two major holidays in one week! The Seder is the focus for Passover. The Hebrew word Seder translates to "order". (One course of dinner follows another in a prescribed order and one prayer follows another.) Every year, the same food is served … and served … and served. Easter Sunday dinner is the focus for Easter. The Easter meal is often eaten at brunch, probably because it always falls on Sunday. In our culture, we put the word "Sunday" together with "brunch". We often go out after a service.

There are, of course, also Easter dinners. I'm sure we all know what Christmas dinners are like.

3. Birthday Parties

- What's the first thing you think of when you think of a birthday party? I sincerely doubt you think of asparagus. There's an old superstition that tells us it's *unlucky not to share in a birthday cake.* While I doubt this means you'll die if you don't have a piece of cake, it's fun to take a piece, and you can feel loving when you partake with the birthday boy/girl, thus contributing to their joy.
- *Note that a small forkful fulfills your obligation,* and you can sing just as loudly as if you had a whole wedge of cake. When they say piece, they don't mention the size.

4. Weddings, Bar Mitzvahs, Christenings, etc.

- I separate weddings and birthday parties because weddings often extend for a longer period of time than most birthday parties. Weddings may involve more than one day of eating. Aside from the actual ceremony, most of the activity is eating.
- If you're part of the wedding party, you often have a rehearsal dinner as well.
- At each seating and cocktail reception, it can be fun to *eye the hors d'oeuvres for a while and make your choices before filling your plate.* This is also an excellent time to socialize. Finding the veggies that are beneficial to you is a good idea. They usually have a vegetable dish. A little dip won't kill you at a wedding. Just a drop on, say, a carrot can make you feel like you're really munching away. Keeping a glass of water

in your hand can help too. Actually, a glass or two (not five glasses at once) of red wine is beneficial for some people. Check and see which wines—if any—are good for you. Red wine is healthy for many people.

5. Girls'/Boys' Night Out

- Now that we're living longer and better, even those who are living with spouses or significant others will often be invited to join a girls' or boys' night out. I've experienced that the psychology of going out with a gang, especially when another person set up the evening, can have little twists to it.
- If you're at a girls' night out, remember to breathe. Talk calmly to yourself and give yourself permission to set your boundaries. I understand that you want to be considered a team player, and you want to be liked by the rest of the group. That said, the practice of ordering dishes for everyone and then having everyone share the orders can invade your freedom. You very often don't get to choose the foods that are best for you. This can be especially troublesome if the person who organized the evening doesn't have (or doesn't think they have) the same food needs you do.
- Planning what's on the table is certainly a person's right if you're invited to his or her home for dinner. However, if you're sharing the bill as well as the food, this is a wonderful time for you to practice speaking up for yourself and setting your boundaries.
- Humans often think that "giving ourselves permission" means permission to do or have something that isn't good for us. But it also means giving ourselves permission to do what's great for us!

6. Business Dinners and Dinners Involving Projects We're Involved In

- Industry and national company dinners often involve travel. If you're still working, you may find yourself at a company dinner.
- Some Seniors are still working, even though many have been laid off. . Company dinners may include some people who are over sixty or seventy years of age as well as employees who are in their twenties, thirties, and forties at various levels of a corporate chart. Although the older population has grown greatly unfortunately many seniors and healthy employees who are in their 50s and early 60s have been let go from their jobs or been put on a part time schedule. This is a whole other issue. Ageism has developed on our planet and, certainly, in our country. Years ago, the top levels of the corporate matrix were usually older, and the body of the company was younger. Now the opposite can hold true. The older workers are often on part-time schedules.

  - Please do a "Google search" for "The Radical Age Movement", which was founded by Alice Fisher, who recently retired as Outreach Director for State Senator Liz Krueger. Senator Krueger understood that Alice needed to move on and spend her time building this most important movement. Whatever age you are now, the issue of Ageism will affect you at some point in your life if it isn't curbed. Please let Alice know I directed you to the group.

- You're now likely to see people of different ages at many networking events too. While many networking events are in college clubs and industry clubs, many are also held in restaurants. The clubs usually have dining areas too.

- If the dinner at the event is served buffet style, you can follow the fun method I found. I call it "The Secret Guilty List!" & it's explained after Section 8 in this list.

  By the way, do you have projects you're passionate about? I hope you do! As I said earlier, passion for living and for learning new things will usually inspire you to keep your body in shape.

7. Professional Sports Events

- "Take me out to the ball game. Take me out with the crowd." It can really be fun to go to a game with one of more fans. It's the second line of that song that can prove interesting for people who have their minimum quantity lists. "Buy me some peanuts or crackerjacks. I don't care if I never get back!"
- I could imaging that song including custard and sausage and bubbling six-packs and all sorts of stadium food. Food has become an important revenue stream for stadiums. In a way, this helps us. While they used to just have the concession stands, there is now more choice and some "real" food available.
- Note, however, that many people link sports with beer and heavier snacks. There is no uniformity in how revenue from food is disbursed in stadiums, so there's no law against bringing in your own food. You'll read more about this in chapter 13.
- Etiquette at the ballpark often includes, "Here—take a bite." You can make the kind person who's offering feel great by smiling and gently patting the back of his/her hand. *You're not required to bite.*

- Being at the ball field also requires breathing and making your own decisions about what to eat. It's easy to want to please your partner or group and eat traditional sports food, which is what I used to call guy food. I don't think I have to list the foods.

8. Music Rooms, Cabarets, and Clubs That Have Minimum Food and Beverage Charges

I've added this situation to the seven that were in my first book. I realize that some people are surprised when they see there is a minimum charge, although the clubs almost always list that if it's something they practice. Note that the clubs need to have these minimum charges because the entrance fee is usually low, and the entrance fee is how the club pays the performer. In order for the club to stay in business, it needs to charge a minimum for drinks and snacks.

Some people mistakenly feel that this minimum obliges them to have an alcoholic beverage. Please note that if alcoholic beverages aren't healthy for you, you are in no way obliged to order one. All clubs have choices of soft drinks. By the way, unless you have certain specific conditions, red wine is very healthy for people with blood type A and super beneficial for certain blood types. The worst that red wine is rated for any specific blood type is "neutral." I don't see any "harmful" listing for it. However, you don't have to order even wine. I think that all cabaret rooms have juice. The drinks and foods on the menu in cabaret rooms aren't very expensive, and they're not usually large portions. At a supper club, you may be able to order a whole dinner.

By the way, the minimum usually refers to drinks. However, there are a few clubs that require a minimum food purchase. If you can, check out the menu before you go to the show. You may not have much time to look at it otherwise. You may find it online. If there's nothing on the menu that's healthy for you, let the club know. You might be helping the establishment. They could let people know that they care about their patrons and want to serve food that's known to be healthy. Only a few people know what's truly best for them.

Check out any club you plan to go to beforehand so you're aware of any minimums you may be charged. Life is simpler when you know what you want to order when you enter a club. It's nice to have something to munch on and to drink while watching a cabaret show.

Once you know the foods that are best for you, you can check out what any menu has on it and choose whether or not to eat it beforehand.

How do I choose foods that help me achieve my dreams of fitness in these situations? Let's take it step by step.

Here's what helped me: *The Secret "Guilty"Llist!*

Note: *you* are never the guilty party!

I formed my own secret "guilty" list! (Guilty List? What is Bobbie talking about?) I highly advise that you do the same!

In one of my workshops, I shared an experience I had while serving on a jury. I realized I could use the concept I derived from that jury experience to help me not eat foods that don't serve me!

I was on a jury about a decade ago and got on one simple, short case. We made the decision in record time because we had a brilliant jury foreman. The penalty for the case wasn't life threatening for the defendant. He was videotaped taking items from a counter at Bloomingdales. We went back into the jury room, and our foreman immediately said, "I know we all feel for the poor man who was videoed. He may have needed the items ... and ... before we discuss the case, let's see how many of us suspect that the plaintiff is guilty of taking the items in question." We all raised our hands. Then we did discuss the case. In this country, thankfully, we have a fair system. I was touched by with the kindness of all on the jury. It took us only ten minutes to reach a verdict. After all, we clearly saw him take the items. Did we feel sorry for him? Yes. Did he take the items? Yes.

What does this have to do with food? I think *we know pretty quickly after we've set up our mini-Qs which foods are "guilty" for us.* In chapter 6, you looked at your body's history with different foods. You were able to see which foods worked better for you in terms of energy, digestion, and nourishment. We spoke of foods that satiated your hunger for long periods of time. The top food choices in the latter group were those that also had great nourishment value.

You don't have to feel that you're giving up foods that aren't great for you—but rather that you're sentencing them to the guilty pile. They're lucky that you let them get away with murder! At this point, they may still taste delicious. However, after some time in the guilty pile, you might find that your taste for them changes. Mine certainly did! I find it impossible to bite into certain foods I used to love! I think I could only bite into a hot pastrami sandwich now if my life truly depended on it! *You're not denying yourself* this way. You're giving a *"yes"* to these foods being guilty. It's not, "No, I can't have you," but rather, "Yes! I'm saying you're guilty."

CHAPTER 12

Seven Tips for Appearing Slimmer/ Fuller While Dropping/Adding Pounds

I was certified in image consulting by Image Consultants International in the early nineties. I teach, what I call, Dress to Get "YES!" seminars, in which I analyze each participant's color(s) and style(s), and I also teach color psychology workshops. Finding the right clothes for me and the right makeup and hairdo has been a passion of mine since I can remember. I think I instinctively knew, since early childhood, that the way people presented themselves to others affected the responses they got from others. Of course, what I'm calling instinct may have been the influence of my dad, who was a fashion enthusiast. He would have gone into the men's clothing business after he graduated from college in 1928 had the Great Depression not hit in 1929.

I also care about sharing what I've learned about keeping in shape with you. I was not in good shape when I was in my early sixties and I realized I had to do something about that. I did a huge amount of research and came up with what helped me get fit. As you know, this book is about helping you find the methods that best work for you and places you can check out, so you can put together a way for you to be as fit as you possibly can. While you're doing that, I'll give you some tips about style that can help your appearance while you're on your way and when you've reached your fitness goals. The links to my site and my blog are at the end of this book. You'll find a free Monthly Image Tip on the site and tips on the blog. We've already discussed the benefits of knowing what your style is. These tips are about choosing clothes (in your style) that will camouflage your body's imperfections and will help you look better while you're following your plan to get it into it's optimum shape. These tips can also help you throughout your life. This is a sneak peek from a future book I plan to write.

1. Trick the viewer's eye—appear slimmer/fuller while you're dropping/adding pounds.

If you're in the process of dropping pounds, here are some tips:

- Wear an outfit that doesn't hug you (for jacket length, etc., see number four below) in one of the dark neutral colors from the palette(s) that harmonizes with your skin tone (see number two).
- Wear a long, narrow, lightweight scarf in one of your lightest (bright could work too) colors tied around your neck and let it hang as long as the length can be down the center of your body. The light stripe, as it were, brings the viewer's eye to the center of your body, and the person focuses on the long, narrow stripe, so the rest of your body receives less focus. A long, long, strand of small (for example) pearls can achieve the same effect. A man's suit is designed like this. When you wear a light shirt and tie in the middle of a dark suit, it brings the eye in. In cool weather, he can wear a thin, light-colored muffler and let it hang down the center of his body.

- Note that if your face is long, you won't want the pearls to be very long. In this case, they would suit you better if they were just a bit longer than a choker. If your neck is tight and smooth, you could wear a choker to shorten the appearance of your long face.

- Look for formal wear that's a solid color. Choose a darker color within your palette. You may have a combination of palettes to choose from. Know your style (or combination of styles). You can use your own unique style to help you.
- Example: for a woman who is dramatic in style, a dark dress or jacket with an asymmetrical stripe going from one shoulder to the opposite hip can be slenderizing and dramatic.
- If you have a scrawny body and you're trying to add pounds, the opposite of what I said above holds. Wear light colors toward the outside of your body to widen you to the viewer's eye. Wearing too tight clothing (even though you can) will emphasize scrawniness. Clothing that is too loose can make you look too thin. Look for outfits that are neither tight nor loose. Take your time choosing clothing. If you can't find clothes that fit you perfectly, a good tailor is a good investment. Being too thin or being too heavy can be aging.
- Note: <u>I'm trying to find another word for "aging."</u> I think being older is a good thing. The word should have something to do with health and vitality. We need to change our vocabulary so that age isn't taken negatively.

2. Know your unique color palette(s) and style(s). It will be a great help to you.

- If you haven't already had your color palette(s) and style(s) analyzed by an expert, do so. If you're in the NYC area, I'd be happy to work with you. Bring a proof of purchase of the book, and you'll get a 10 percent discount on any service I provide. If you live elsewhere, contact me, and I'll do my best to find a good image consultant in your area. Go to my website, www.bobbiehorowitz.com, click on Contact, and let me know you need information. I'll get in touch with you, and we'll discuss your needs, and I'll let you know the cost of the services you require. I can help you pinpoint your style through an inexpensive telephone consultation. You'll need to send me a few pictures of yourself for this. I'd need to have an appointment with you in person to analyze your colors. I hold classes and conduct private consultations. You'll get as much time as is required for an individual analysis. The classes cost less. As I said, I'll recommend someone in your area if you can't get to New York City.

- It's so important to know your own unique palette(s) and style(s) because it affects the way people subliminally perceive you. On my site, you'll see a painting by Picasso in two different frames. I think you'll find it clear that in one frame you immediately "get" what the painting is telling you, and in the other, it takes a minute or two to figure it out. What's going on in the viewer's mind is going on subliminally. They're not aware it's happening.

- When the style, or combination of styles, you wear harmonizes with your body and facial attributes and your personality, people will "get" who you are within the first thirty seconds of meeting you. Please note that the other party has no idea his/her understanding is based on your appearance. This is all subliminal! It's where art and science meet. Packaging companies know this! Why shouldn't you?

- In addition to conveying your personality, when the colors you're wearing harmonize with your skin tone, you'll appear more rested. You'll have fewer facial lines, dark circles under your eyes will lessen, and your skin will appear clearer.

3. Check your outfit out by looking in the mirror.

- I bet you're thinking, *Duh! Everyone knows to look in the mirror!* I notice, however, that many people miss certain things.
- If possible, install a full-length mirror somewhere in your home.
- Be sure to look at all the different views of yourself in any outfit. After you look straight ahead, turn to each side. You'd be amazed at how many extremely overweight performers I see go on stage in stretch fabric gowns—or, for men, trousers—and don't realize that their tummy is protruding or their derriere looks uneven or floppy. What happens then is that the audience isn't paying attention to the performance. They're looking at the performer's figure whether or not they realize they are.
- Bring a hand mirror with you so you can see the reflection of the back of your outfit. Looking into two full mirrors that reflect into each other is the best way to look at yourself. I realize this isn't always possible to do.
- Know that the mirror is merely a reflection of how you appear right now. That appearance will change when you do. There is nothing real in the mirror. It's just a reflection of what you've chosen.

4. Know your body proportions.

- If you possibly can, have a trained image consultant analyze them with you.
- Check the lengthwise proportion of your torso to your legs.
- If your legs look short (many men look like they're standing in a hole when their legs are shorter than their torsos), shortening your jacket can make a distinctive difference and vice versa.

- If you are a man and you're fairly short, it is best to wear trousers that have no cuffs. If you are very tall, wear cuffed trousers.

- Check the width of your shoulders as compared to the width of your hips. Both men and women can appear to have slimmed down their hips by simply adding shoulder pads to balance their shoulders to their hips. You won't want to overdo it. The goal is balance.

- Check out any other body disproportions you may have. If you have a hunching curve in your back, wearing a jacket with a larger and structured collar and somewhat structured shoulders with a back that doesn't cling can help. You can buy a slightly larger jacket and have a tailor take in the front if necessary. For women and men, unless your legs are quite a bit shorter than your torso, it's also a good idea for your jacket to be long enough to reach your derriere, so that it doesn't stand away from your body and emphasize the spine curve. If you have a disability or if you are confined to a wheelchair, wear the bright colors of your palette near your face to bring joy to it. This is true for people show aren't disabled also. The same ideas about proportion apply to you. If you have limited or no vision, it would be great if you can have someone come in and organize your closet in terms of colors, etc. and put different shaped tags on the hangers—with the shape linked to a color or a style, so you can find things more easily. People who are colorblind would be serviced by having their closets organized by color and having tags with the colors written on them on the hangers. It's usually just a few colors that aren't distinguished, and it usually occurs in men.

5. Check out the shape of your eyeglass or sunglass frames.

- If your face is long and thin, you'll look younger and bouncier with frames that broaden your eye area and, therefore, help your face to look less long. You won't want the frames to be too thin. A round frame can work in this case if the frame for each eye is a wide circle and it's not too narrow at the nose area.

- The opposite of the above will be true if your face is round. You wouldn't want round glasses. You wouldn't want the frames themselves to be too thin because that would draw attention to the size of your face. A middle-sized pair that's oblong (side to side) would work well.

6. Check out your shoes.

- This may sound ridiculously obvious, but it is always beneficial to pay attention to any pain you may be having as a result of wearing less than well-fitting shoes. When. ou walk in pain, you look less healthy and less attractive. Different people need different amounts of support in different areas of their feet. I had foot surgery about a decade ago, and I had to go from being a three-inch heel wearer to a wearer of flats. Help! Thankfully I found a wonderful pair of shoes that I get in every color. I've even had them died to a metallic gold hue! Heel height, of course, refers more to women's shoes than men's. However, I know men who didn't realize that their feet didn't have to hurt until they went to a store that could cater to their needs.

- If possible, find a shoe store with an in-house orthopedist. The shoes are often quite expensive. However, when you consider the cost-per-wearing factor, they can be well worth it. They're making many more shoes for people with orthopedic concerns than they did when I was a kid. It also helps to have your shoes and socks or stockings have colors as close in color to the rest of your outfit as possible.

- Orthotics can be a major help. Your heels may pronate (lean) inward or outward. You may have fallen arches. Many foot conditions, like those I've mentioned can be helped by wearing orthotics. Note, that after you body has been used to walking a certain way for many years, these shoes may take some getting used to. There is a product that restores the glutathione (the body's key protein and antioxidant, which has an anti-inflammatory component to it. It's listed in my recommendations. At any rate, you deserve to be comfortable.

- Unless you're a woman who has long, slender calves and thighs, you'll look better with one color going from your waist to the floor. Your skirt might have a line going down it, asymmetrically, but one color is usually more flattering when you're working toward being your slender, healthy self. Again, having shoes that blend into your outfit, color-wise, helps you look sleek.

7. Check out your hairstyle.

- The hairstyle you choose can do a lot to help you appear trimmed down or fill out your face.
- The texture of your hair is part of what makes up your style. You can use your hair to benefit the shape of your face and, to some extent, the way your body appears to others.
- For example, my face is longish—thinner than it is wide— and I have defined cheekbones, a narrow chin, full lips, and a long neck. It's what image consultants call a dramatic shape with a touch of natural thrown in. A dramatic shape will most often go with smooth, somewhat fine, shiny hair. The texture of my hair is natural. It goes with my autumnal coloring. It's thick, rough, and wavy. It's curlier

when it's short. I wear it mid-length. I have to keep it very moisturized. It helps me balance the shape of my face since I can get width out of it. I pick a hairstyle with width to it. I like the 1940s look because my style is closest to that we associate with the war years (WWII).

- In our culture, an oval face is often considered the thing to aim for. It's what we image consultants would call a classic style of face. By the way, there is no one shape of face that's better than any other shape. If you wish to exaggerate the shape of the face you have, that's fine with me. It will work if you have the personality that goes with it. Your personality usually mirrors aspects of your personal style. That said, women and men alike can use their hair to balance their faces. It can give us what we've come to consider a more pleasing shape.

- If you have a very round face, you can choose a hairdo that diagonally sweeps across your face. You might want your hair to be a bit longer. This will cut across the roundness and make your face appear more oval shaped.

- Baldness for men is a choice that works well with many face shapes. It adds a slightly dramatic touch, but it fits with any style. It's gotten much more acceptable, even fashionable in recent years.

- I've seen men in great hairpieces. However, more often than not, I see the hairpiece walk into the room before the man. It's best to have a consultation with an image consultant and/or go to a hairdresser who really knows the image business and how to work with a hairpiece.

- I've seen some wonderful wigs for women whose hair may be thinning naturally or due to medication. Choose the wig as you'd choose your hair. Take it to your hairdresser to be trimmed, shaped for you, and/or thinned if needed. Check that the color is in your palette.

CHAPTER 13

Keep Shinin', _____'s Star

(Your Name)

Welcome to the Wow Galaxy! You're twinkling and bright. You're a true work of art. Now that you've revealed yourself, it's time to write a description of yourself as the star you truly are!

As I've previously said, I find the actual act of writing stimulating, and writing helps me remember the thought and the image that was in my brain when I had the thought. Photos can help too. It's easy to forget the specifics of what you were thinking or truly seeing at any given moment. In this case, you'll want to keep the description of you, as the star you truly are, in your brain.

Use whatever means works for you. This way you'll be able to take stock in the future to see if you're still allowing yourself to continually physically appear as "you the star." After you've been around for a while without the excess surrounding your true self, you'll find it easier to continually be that star.

Here's a list of items you may want to check out at varying time intervals:

Weight: _____

I suggest you weigh yourself on the same scale every morning when you get up, before you have anything to drink or eat. If you're travelling, try to find a scale where you're staying. Don't go crazy if there isn't one. It's not going to make a huge difference in your life. It's just nice to see that you're on target.

Note: Your scale may show an increase of a pound or two some days and a loss on some days. Just keep track over time to see you're within a couple of pounds of your true weight. You may still have liquid in your system. Other factors affect your exact weight from day to day. If you see the scale go up more than two or three pounds on any day, spend a day eating those organic vegetables and fruits that are highly beneficial for you and a handful of nuts, and drink a lot of water. Or do a cleanse day (see my recommendations) in the near future.

Waist measurement: _____
Chest measurement: _____
Hips measurement: _____

You can take your waist, chest, and hip measurements, or better yet, notice how your clothes are fitting. My favorite way to see what's happening is to check out how my clothes are fitting. I had seemingly miraculous happenings since I dropped weight. *I needed to have my clothes taken in three times!* The first time was after I dropped about thirty pounds. I could have had them taken in before that, but I wanted to keep dropping pounds and didn't want to feel comfortable until I did. I didn't realize I could drop more than thirty pounds! After I dropped an additional thirteen pounds - I had them taken in again. Then came the surprise! After about nine months I needed to alter my clothes yet again … and … then again - because my weight shifted - and a few things needed additional minor alterations. *My weight had been redistributed from fat to muscle!* The mini-Qs I used to drop and now to maintain my weight also helped me build muscle. You can read about it under my recommendations. The products I mention work for most people. You need to decide if it's something that would work for you. I would try them out and then make your decision.

Even the brightest stars in the heavens appear clouded over to the planets spinning around them now and again, so there's no need to beat yourself up if one morning you get on the scale and see some extra "stone" around you, the perfect statue. Don't beat yourself up; however get back on track to being the size that's best for you.

PART III
Bobbie's Plan for Bobbie

(Your Plan Will Be for You)

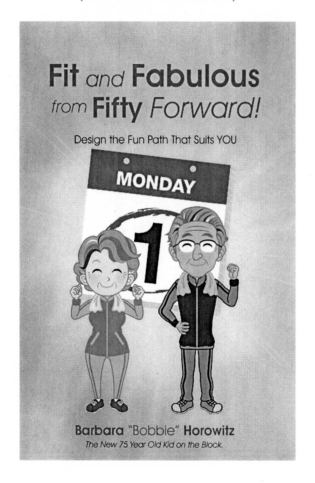

Fit *and* **Fabulous**
from **Fifty** *Forward!*

Design the Fun Path That Suits YOU

MONDAY
1

Barbara "Bobbie" Horowitz
The New 75 Year Old Kid on the Block.

CHAPTER 14

Bobbie's "Mini-Qs" (i.e., Get-to-Dos) for Nourishment

(In case you'd like to know how I dropped weight and what I continue to do now to keep it off.)

To repeat: *While the process of setting up one's get-to-dos is the same for everyone, the specific choices made by each person depend on the biological needs of that person. You'll choose the specific choices for your body's needs. We've discussed how you can find out the most beneficial foods for you.*

The most surprising thing happened to me! No joke! Now, as I told you before, I truly do not miss or even think about the foods that I found out I should avoid.

Take a look at the procedure I used to set up what I do and the products I use and see if you think any of it can work for you. It may save you some time or, at least give you a starting point. Remember, I've named my daily get-to-dos my mini-Qs (mini represents the minimum quantity of each to-do that I get to do each day). Note that saying *get* to do gives them a positive connotation. Saying minimum lets me breathe. It's not that much of anything! I can do it!

I turned seventy-five years of age on May 22, 2015 and I weigh 126 pounds! I've maintained a weight of 126 pounds for about eleven years. I'm now about 5'5&1/2" tall. I've lost two inches of height over the past 15 years, so I guess I actually weigh a bit more per inch of height than I did when I first lost the pounds.

I bet if I knew what I know now when I was in my twenties, thirties, and forties, I wouldn't have lost that height.

My muscles are much more solid now than when I was young. I hardly ever get a cold and I have great and mostly stable energy! All my medical readings are now "near poifect!," as we would have said in Brooklyn. I was taking a few pharmaceuticals in my fifties and early to mid-sixties. When I wrote the first edition of this book, I took only one

Some Background

In high school, I was sad about my weight—although, looking back, in high school I wasn't really fat! I was fat for a few years, as a preteen. That preteen image we have of ourselves is often hard to shake. *They announced my weight—<u>out loud</u>—in a classroom filled with the girls and boys in both the first grade and the fifth grade! When I was in the fifth grade, I was eleven years old and weighed 165 pounds! Aaaah!*

This memory holds a place in one of the comedy songs I've written about life in New York—Brooklyn in particular. In high school, I was 5 feet, 7¾ inches tall and weighed 146 pounds. I wasn't thin, but I was not really fat either. I lost ten pounds naturally between junior high and high school. But I wasn't ever the one who'd make the cheerleaders. That was probably because I held the image of "fat" in my mind. I was elected president of New Utrecht High School, but that wasn't an ego trip for me. Being a cheerleader would have been. Cheerleaders were the gorgeous girls who were slim and wore short cheerleading skirts! When I moved away from my family and into my dorm at Cornell, I became very weight conscious. I lost thirteen pounds freshman semester as a result of leaving home and eating like Middle America ate in the 1950s (before McDonald's). I admit to probably having undiagnosed borderline anorexia through my twenties. My mom was nervous for me. I did catch germs that were going around in those days, and my back often hurt. I now weigh almost as little as I did in the anorexia days, but I'm solid. I rarely get a cold, and I feel great!

In my late fifties and early sixties, I was producing theater. One was a musical, *The Betrayal of Nora Blake* in London and West Palm Beach, and one was an awards event. I was co-executive producer of Drama Desk Awards in 1999 and 2000 and associate producer in 2001. At the same time, I was setting up the Times Square Group, a nonprofit arts-in-education company that brought hands-on theatrical programs into New York City high schools and middle schools. Although this was a very exciting and fulfilling time in my life, there was also a lot of tension involved with each project. I was also dealing with my mother's dementia and finally her passing. Two years prior to my mom's passing, my wonderful baby sister passed from hepatitis caused by a bad blood transfusion during a surgical procedure thirty years before. They didn't know to screen blood for hepatitis then. You can say what happened was life. I mentioned her in chapter 2. It was a productive and, at the same time, very intense and stressful period for me. With almost all of my family gone, I felt it was all up to me. I was the one who would have to see to it that I survived and that my son did well. Have you felt like that? You may very well have. In any case, take a deep breath and *be thankful.* Either way, *be thankful!* It's all a process. Thankfully, my spiritual counselor and Reiki teacher, Barbara Van Diest, dared to tell me that I was looking much more haggard and heavy than I had to. Thus, I began my trip back to being slender and to being healthier than I think I've ever been.

A good example of why you should keep checking the news!

Once again, I found out new information.

We were ready to go to print with my first book. We were just waiting for the book's ISBN number. Bingo! A few days before we got it, my doctor suggested that I see a specialist for a test. It was a checkup for a slight medical condition that made me a little uncomfortable after having had surgery for uterine cancer about five years before my first book came out (almost nine years ago now). Thankfully, the test showed I was fine. The specialist suggested that I add soy to my diet to help lubricate the lining of my bladder. Wow! As you'll see below, I'd started with products from Dr. D'Adamo. These were soy based. They were pure and organic soy. Be sure to check your products. Soy is beneficial for blood type A Positive, which I am. I used his soy protein powder. I continued to follow and enjoy the food choices for blood type A. I totally trusted Dr. D'Adamo, but reports came out that soy could encourage certain cancers. So I cut down on soy and stopped using his soy protein powder. That's when I was introduced to Isagenix, which uses whey protein from a special ecosystem in New Zealand. I have to watch whey, but this amount seemed okay for me. They've since come out with nondairy shakes that work very well for me. While instinctively feeling that I could eat soy too, I avoided it because I'd heard it was sprayed with unnatural substances. I just ate a little organic edamame now and then and soymilk in my coffee. Are you still with me?

About four years ago, I started seeing articles stating that soy can be grown organically and actually help prevent certain cancers! So, after the specialist told me to eat soy, I asked two other doctors about soy and cancer, and I got the full "go ahead."

Again, I like to get opinions from three different experts in a field before making a decision about something that's been questionable. Note: when it comes to soy, it's important to be certain that any product you're going to eat that's made from American soybeans is organic and hasn't in any way been genetically altered.

Why is this important for you? This substantiates the value of revising your get-to-dos when needed and getting your doctors' opinions. You can then redesign your daily living to include the better option. Designing your own best way to eat and move and, in truth, do anything necessitates keeping aware of life around you. Do some research and then trust yourself. Things you've always wanted might just start showing up! I will place any new things I find out on my website for you.

I began my rejuvenation by just following the advice I got from Dr. Peter D'Adamo about eating for my blood type. I began dropping pounds. I was very happy. A year or so after meeting Dr. D'Adamo's staff, I was introduced to Isagenix and did what was called a nine-day cleanse. It was the only plan they had in November 2003 when I was introduced to the company. It was intense, but I was committed and completed it with a friend. I dropped eleven pounds in nine days! Then I followed what they call their thirty-day plan for about six months, and then I weighed 126 pounds, and I never went back. I didn't yet have my mini-Q concept. I found this plan made my life easier. Blending was simpler than cooking for me, and I could still go out for a meal every day. Then I started to play with the shakes, adding healthy berries, pine nuts, etc. I still often have two Isagenix meals a day. I enjoy them, and I feel great. See if it works for you. Note that the products are improved when new things are found out.

Note: After using Isagenix for several years I discovered that "whey protein" wasn't the best for me and that I should avoid it when possible.

We keep learning as science makes new discoveries. Now I use the Isagenix protein powders that are "whey free" or contain very little weigh. I know their whey is, at least, denatured and carefully processed.

If the idea of mini-Qs (get-to-dos) hadn't hit me in the head, I'm not sure I'd have kept the weight away from me. I do still believe in the cleanse idea, especially in the beginning stages of wanting to change your weight. I've also seen many people who were helped by products stop using those products that benefitted them. The mini-Qs are how and why I stick with what works for me, and they're helping others stay slim, sexy, and healthy too.

I was introduced to MAX International in January 2010. The company's product devisor had close ties with the Mayo Clinic. I still take some of their supplements that are wonderful for me and complement the other supplements I take. *Be careful not to double on some contents when you choose supplements from more than one company.

I learned about what they call "Nightshade Vegetables" from Dr. D'Adamo. Within about four months after stopping eating them my joint pain began to subside, and within a year, the bumps on my index finger knuckles were down significantly. I now have no bumps and no pain!
You can find out what vegetables these are by searching the Internet for "Nightshade Vegetables". If you don't now know about them you may be surprised to find out which they are. They are not "bad" in and of themselves and there are some who say they don't affect osteoarthritis pain. Not eating them certainly stopped my pain when medications didn't. All I can say is: "I'm thrilled to not be taking medications for my pain and I'm thrilled for having NO pain since I've avoided Nightshades.

Note that some of the items in the following groups of "mini-Qs" (as I've named my plan) are different from those mentioned in my original book, "Find your mini-Qs". As my body and system changed and as new products cam out I changed s few of those I'd been taking.

It's a good idea to always keep up with what's being discovered. Health knowledge is one area of knowledge that's expanded greatly in recent years and keeps expanding. We can all be very grateful for this.

My Morning Food Mini-Qs

1. I begin each day with a simple little cleanse and energy boost.

> I squeeze half a lemon into a half cup of warm water. I add one ounce of Isagenix Cleanse for Life.nd one ounce of Isagenix Ionix Supreme to my morning Harvest Berry flavored shake. That flavor doesn't have dairy in it.

> I drink 4–8 ounces of deacidified water.

2. I then take the following supplements (I know this can look like a lot. I think of them as food.):

a. One Isagenix Natural Accelerator
b. One IsaOmega fatty-acids capsule
c. One Max N-Fuze vitamins with nano-activators
d. Three Isagenix Joint Support tablets
e. One cranberry tablet (I've had surgery for uterine cancer, and this is very helpful for me. This isn't medicine. Ask your doctor about it. It helps keep away urinary problems. You can get it in most drugstores.)
f. One or two MAX ONE capsules. They said people should take one capsule twice a day. These contain Glutathione.

> Note: When I asked them if more could hurt – they have incredible benefits, especially for someone like me and they didn't seem to have anything that could be harmful in

them, I was told that several people, especially people who are older, take many more and do well. I usually take two before breakfast and two before lunch.

Note: I have these about fifteen minutes before breakfast. I do my face exercises after taking these supplements.

3. Breakfast at home is the same almost every day.

a. To repeat: I mix an Isagenix shake (usually Berry Harvest). I blend it with less water than called for, and I make up the difference with chopped ice. I get it really thick, like ice cream. It has great consistency for my taste. It was designed to be a shake. I won't get the company angry when I say I make it my way. I've already told them play with the consistency.

b. Then I usually add, depending on the flavor shake I've chosen, a handful each of walnuts and "Kind" cereal, in flavors with ingredients that are good for my blood type, for crunch and the benefits they have for me. In addition to many health-food stores, many supermarkets now carry this brand. If you can't find this brand ask a nutritionist you trust what companies make good cereal products you can use instead.

c. One cup of organic coffee with just a little (organic) vanilla Soy Milk. I use a little stevia powder to sweeten it. It did take me a while to find a brand of stevia I liked. It's a naturally grown plant that doesn't have calories. I had trouble finding a brand with a flavor I like. I love Sweet Leaf (in the concentrated form)—in the container.

d. Either lunch or dinner can be a regular meal, because I often have food at meetings or music performances.

4. Lunch or dinner at home is almost the same every day.

    a. Note that my lunch supplements are:
- One or two MAXONE capsules. They said people should take one capsule twice a day. I mentioned why I often take two in the Breakfast listing.
- One Isagenix Accelerator capsule
- One cranberry tablet

    b. I'll make a shake from one of the soup flavors. I like it thick, as I like my breakfast shake. I like it cold and not warm like soup usually is. You can decide for yourself.

    c. I get to add veggies to this. I put in edamame (soy beans) and packaged veggies like broccoli slaw or carrots and broccoli spears cut up, chopped onions, pine nuts, and any other fun veggies I find in the supermarket that are good for my type. I like things crunchy and raw. To repeat: you may cook your food if you prefer it that way.

    d. I have a cup of organic green tea with just a little organic stevia powder.

Remember that you follow what works for you and what you like. This is about you!

5. Breakfast or lunch or dinner on the run can be an Isagenix bar.

6. If I'm meeting someone for breakfast, I almost always order the following:

    a. An egg-white omelet with spinach and/or broccoli, with mozzarella or goat cheese.

    b. I'll eat the crust of a piece of rye toast or the top of a toasted oat muffin, if the restaurant has an oat muffin.

    c. I carry my own stevia. I prefer the taste of stevia packaged in the container. I find the packets change the taste to me.

d. I have one cup of coffee. I'll sometimes order a refill when the waiter comes around, with a drop of cream (if they have it) or Half & Half. If they have soymilk, I'll choose that. I hardly ever use milk.

> Note: The doctor who examined me at Dr. D'Adamo's office told me it was best for me to avoid plain milk and especially to avoid skim milk. Surprised? So was I. It has to do with "lectins". Who knew?

> Note: I always say "Guilty!" to nightshades like potatoes and tomatoes or peppers, eggplant, chickpeas, paprika, and chili because they heighten osteoarthritis.

6. This is what I have for a midmorning snack:

1. If I'm hungry, I'll have a half (which sometimes becomes a whole) plum or a peach. Plums are very beneficial for me. You can check to see which fruits and veggies are most beneficial for you. I may also have an Isagenix Fibre Snack. I always need to make sure I'm eliminating properly and these are a great source of fibre.

7. Dinner or lunch out can be challenging.

> This can prove a challenge, especially if I'm in one of the possible "Strike-Out situations" I mentioned.

> In an American or continental restaurant, I almost always order a green salad, sautéed salmon, and a side of broccoli rabe if the restaurant has it. (I just happen to love it!) I may order a fruit cup for dessert, if everyone is having dessert, and I give away the fruits that aren't good for my blood type. Japanese restaurants are very easy, as are Chinese and

Thai restaurants, unless they're Sichuan. Then I need to say, "Guilty!" to the spicy peppers. Middle Eastern restaurants can prove a challenge to me due to the chickpeas, eggplant, and other nightshade veggies that are so often used. However, I can usually find something that works for me in any kind of restaurant.

Note: Choose the foods that are beneficial for you.

Note two: **Can you tell I'm having fun with this? I really am!** I'm in charge of any menu that's placed in front of me. I tell the waiter to prepare me feeling like I'm in a Jackie Mason sketch! Everybody gets a laugh!

8. My bedtime supplements are the following:

   a. An omega fatty-acids capsule
   b. An IsaFlush capsule
   c. One cranberry tablet
   d. One yeast-fighting tablet (I take only one of these per day in the evening.)

CHAPTER 15

Bobbie's Mini-Qs (Get-to-dos) for Exercise – You can name yours

My Daily Mini-Q of Walking One and One Half Miles

In the past few months, I've actually been adding blocks, but I don't want it to feel as though I must do them every day—yet. I may add them in a month or so if I continue walking as many blocks as I have been lately.

I'm sharing this with you because I want you to know you can lead your mind to believe that what you're doing each day is simple. I'm almost always over "Q" (my minimum quota, in case you forgot the term)) for the day! I walk outdoors during the day if the weather is good. I often do the thirty-block walk in one go. Sometimes I divide it up, depending on my chores for the day. If the weather is inclement, I go up to my gym and walk the track, usually in two sets, doing fifteen to twenty blocks in the morning. (One and a half times around the track equals a city block.) I do the additional blocks I need in order to fill my mini-Q later in the day or in the evening, depending on my schedule. If the weather becomes nice, I can complete the second round outdoors.

My Daily Morning Exercise "Mini-Qs"

I do a series of isometric exercises a every morning and one or two additional exercises (when I remember) on the bus. I usually do my isometric facial exercises. I exercise my mouth and chin area while watching the Weather Channel report - before I go to bed Then I don't have to think about them if I need to rush out in the morning. I know you're supposed to leave a day of rest from exercise once a week. If I do rest, it's usually on Sunday morning. Again, I usually do most of these exercises before I even leave my bedroom. I cheer when I can go to the kitchen, take my supplements, and have my morning shake, knowing I've completed my indoor daily exercise mini-Qs! Yay!

Shhh! I've recently begun sneaking a couple of my body exercises before I go to bed at night and count them done for the next morning - in order to have even less to do in the morning.

Note: These may not be right for everyone. The Mayo Clinic has noted that: "It's also important to note that isometric exercises generally aren't recommended for people who have high blood pressure or heart problems." I never had high blood pressure. If anything, mine was a bit low. I used to have high cholesterol but no longer do. Also, for some reason, a fitness doctor that I'd gone to about six years ago prescribed isometrics for me, and they still seem to be working very well for me. This note illustrates the importance of doing your research and asking professionals you trust - to find out what it best for you.

Simple Isometrics

1. With my elbows remaining bent, I hold my hand forward and press my palms together and extend my arms just a bit. Then, while continuing to press my palms together, I tense my stomach muscles

in as hard as I can. I hold this for a count of ten, then another ten, then another ten, and then five. I continue holding the pose and pressing my hands together and tensing my muscles throughout.

When I started, every three days or so I held my arms straight out in front and kept them at shoulder level. Then I put my hands together in prayer position, pressed them together, and then pulled them apart and pulled them down to my sides, clenching them and slowly pulling them outward, tensing the tops and backs of my arms. I was pulling my arms downward and outward at the same time. I now hold this position for a slow count of thirty-five (ten, ten, ten, and five). I now do this exercise, three times in a row, every day. I'm thrilled to report that the flab that was hanging under my upper arms has gotten much tighter! I found that doing this particular exercise three days a week put enough stress on the area for me when I was beginning. Now I'm able to do this every day without any discomfort. Know that you may need to build up the strength to do repetitions every day. I think each person needs to determine if it works for him/her. It would be best for you to discuss this with a physical trainer.

It's a good idea to meet with a few physical trainers before you design your exercise mini-Qs. See who understands that we're not all exactly the same and see who, also, resonates with you. I began with Jonathan Rothschild, and I attribute much of my success to him. He had me working on lifting very heavy weights, very slowly—and only three times lifting each weight, and each time was for a count of thirty. The concept of mini-Q hadn't yet come into my mind yet. I could say my mini-Q for movement was to go to him twice a week for thirty minutes a visit.

I then got to learn about the new machines that were put into my building's health club, and I worked with the great woman, Suzy Sulsona, whose company took over managing the health club. I haven't worked with her for a while but will be working with her again, at least for a while, when you read this. At least every once in a while, it's good to spot check with a trainer you trust.

I bring up all these points to show you that you can go with the possibilities you have near your home and you can revise things when needed.

2. Three or four times a week, I take my shoes or slippers off and bend over as far as I can. I try to press my palms into the floor and hold for a count of twenty. I repeat this at least two times. I happen to have long arms compared to my legs, so it's not all that difficult for me. If your arms are short, you may need to put a box on the floor to lean your hands onto. (My arms may be short – but Not "too short to box with God" though—sorry, I couldn't resist!)

Then, breathing in, I reach my arms up to the ceiling (sky if I'm outdoors) and stretch them as far up as I can, bending my head back and looking up at the ceiling (sky) and letting out a long, strong breath with a "Hah!" or a "Whew!"

3. When I'm sitting on the bus or in a movie or in a coffee shop waiting for someone, I tense my buttocks as strongly as I can and sit with them tensed for a count of thirty. I repeat this twice, and sometimes more times, depending on the time I have and the comfort level of the seat.

My Daily Facial and Neck Exercises

(These work for men and women.)

I can tell you that I don't have many more lines than I did ten years ago, and I've not had plastic surgery. I'd also been developing jowls, which are pretty much gone now. The soft pouch that used to hang under my chin is also pretty much gone now. Yay!

Note: The movements for each of these (except the last) are either a push up or out or a pull down. For each exercise, my underlying muscles are tensing in the opposite direction to the direction in which my fingers are pulling my skin. The counts for each are as follows: ten, then stop; another ten, then stop; another ten, then stop; and finally five, then stop. (10-10-5) This is the same count that I use for my arms and bending exercises.

Forehead, Eyes, and Brows

There are seven exercises for the different areas around your eyes. I hold a piece of tissue against my fingers on each hand so they don't slide on my skin.

1. I spread the fingers of both hands across my forehead and push my fingertips upward, pulling the skin up with them. I concentrate on pulling the muscles in my forehead downward while my index, middle, and ring fingers of each hand are pushing my forehead skin up. I push three lifts to a count of ten each and a fourth lift to a count of five.

2. I spread the fingertips of my left hand under my left brow and the fingertips of my right hand under my right brow and push my fingertips upward, pulling the skin up with them. Similar to the action I use on my forehead, I concentrate on pulling my brow muscles downward while the fingers are pushing up. I push to the above ten/ten/ten/five count.

3. I place the third and fourth fingertips of each hand above my nose and push up, between my eyebrows while pressing down with my forehead. Pushing the muscles against each other causes a tension that firms the muscles. I do the same as in number two, in that I use the ten/ten/ten/five count.

4. Now I take those third and fourth fingertips that are above my nose and between my brows and pull them apart - each toward the outside of my face. At the same time I concentrate on pulling my brows toward the center. This is anther case of having the muscles work against each other, which causes the tension that firms the muscles. Again, I use the ten/ten/ ten/five count.

5. For under my eyes, I place the middle finger of my right hand under my right eye and the middle left finger under my left eye. I then pull my fingers down, while pulling the muscles under my eyes up and fluttering my lids. I use the ten/ten/ten/five count.

6. For the outside corners of my eyes, I place my thumb tips on the outside corners of my eyes, press in, and fast-flutter my eyelashes to the ten/ten/ten/five count.

7. I face forward, and keeping my face facing straight ahead, I gaze up to the ceiling or the sky—as far up as I possibly can. (I can wait and do this one outdoors or on the bus). Do this four times to the same ten/ten/ten/five count. In addition to helping under-eye bags, I think it's helped my vision.

My Jowls and Mouth

There are four exercises for this area. I wear a pair of cotton cloves when doing these.

1. I put my thumbs inside my mouth and press the insides of my thumbs, facing upward, against the insides of my cheeks (right against right and left against left). I then press the index, middle, and ring fingers against the outsides of my cheeks on their respective sides, and I pull down. While I'm pulling down with my fingers, I'm pulling upward with my cheek muscles. I do these using the ten/ten/ten/five count.

2. I put my right-hand thumb on the inside of the lower part of my left jaw and my left hand on the lower part of my right jaw and pull upward while at the same time placing my left-hand index, middle, ring, and pinky fingers on the outside of the lower left part of my face and pull down. I pull four times to the ten/ten/ten/five count. Again, this might sound complicated. When you do it, you'll feel what I mean.

3. I mirror the above exercise on the right jaw area of my face.

4. I place my two index fingers right on the inside corners of my mouth (the right in the right and the left in the left). Then I pull my finger to the sides, stretching my mouth as wide as I can. At the same time, I tense my lips inward. I feel most of the tension on my upper lip. I do that for the ten/ten/ten/five count.

I found it amazing how this helped reduce the little lines on the top of my lip!

5. I put my right index finger inside the right side of my mouth between the upper and lower jaw and my left index finger into my mouth between the upper and lower jaw and squeeze my cheeks and face inward for the ten/ten/ten/five count.

My Neck

1. I make sure I'm sitting or standing up straight and facing forward. I turn my head as far as I can to the left, keeping it on an even level throughout its trip. When my face is as far to the left as it can be, with my back still straight, I lower my chin to my left shoulder as deeply as I can. I lift it up and bring it down slowly (still facing left) for ten counts. Then I bring my face back to the center and do the same thing

for two ten counts and then one five count. Then I do the same on the right side. (It's the old ten/ten/ten/five count.)

Focusing my eyes on something that's a distance past my shoulders helps me to keep my head straight. (This probably sounds more confusing than it actually is.)

2. I clench the center back of the top of my tongue and press it against my upper palette. Then, still pressing my tongue against my upper palette, I bend my head back as far as I can. I hold this for a slow count of ten and do it twice. This is the one that's only two counts of ten. When I think of it, I do this one again in the evening.

Please note that several of the facial exercises were taken from a video that was given to me by the late Barbara Van Diest more than a decade ago. I wish I'd taken a copy of the video so I could order more for clients and friends. I thank the creator of the video—I don't have her name—for all the help she's given me.

Many of my mini-Qs, anyone's "get-to-dos" (to repeat-meaning the minimum repetitions of a task needed to achieve the wanted result), can take patience to get the hang of. I find that so many skills in life depend merely on getting the hang of it! I keep rediscovering this truth. You'd think I'd remember it each time I try something! I'll try a new skill and say, "Oy! Barbara (my birth name is Barbara), you're not meant to do this." Then I think about getting the hang of it, and I learn it fairly easily. *Trust me—you can do it too.*

PART IV
Unsolicited Recommendations and the Wrap-Up

CHAPTER 16

Unsolicited Recommendations

Listen to "The Yes Prayer" by the late Barbara Van Diest every day. Go to https://www.youtube.com/watch?v=rxtoQN_4Ruc

Note: I dedicated the first edition of this book to Barbara, who had such a positive influence on my life and on the lives of so many. It's through Barbara that I met Wayne Dyer and many wonderful spiritual leaders.

Books Plus

1. *Eat Right 4 Your Type* by Dr. Peter D'Adamo
2. *Aging: Fight It with the Blood Type Diet®* by Dr. Peter D'Adamo
3. *The One Minute Manager Gets Fit* by Ken Blanchard, D.W. Edington, Marjorie Blanchard
4. *Wishes Fulfilled* by Dr. Wayne Dyer
5. *The Thought Exchange* by David Friedman
6. *Super You* by Reverend Justin Epstein
7. *The Tapping Solution* by Nickolas Ortner
8. *Refire! Don't Retire* by Ken Blanchard

9. Hay House Publishing—I've found that all the books I've purchased from Hay House Publishing have been helpful.

Live and Web Events

1. Events run by Hay House that deal with your issues are well worth investing in. Some are free. I attended the "I Can Do It" weekend in New York City last summer and found it invaluable. I actually added to my daily fitness mini-Qs as a result of attending. You'll get to meet people you hear about, like Wayne Dyer, Nick Ortner, Carolyn Myss, Dr. Christiane Northrup, etc.

Nickolas Ortner appears at many live events. He was at the Louise Hay "I Can Do It" weekend at the Javits Center in NYC when I attended and I am so glad I attended. I'd worked with his tapping classes online before and had been doing morning tapping meditations for a little over a year before seeing him live. As you can see, I mention him in this book. There are many good programs that derive from ancient practices. People today are discovering new ways of handling physical needs also. To contact Nick Ortner and find out more about EFT (tapping), go to his website: http://www. thetappingsolution.com

The Thought Exchange

David Friedman gives classes in New York City, Connecticut, and a few times a year in Florida. To find out where he is teaching, his site is http://www.thethoughtexchange.com. David is also a well-known composer and was a highly regarded Broadway musical conductor and performance teacher. I take his Inner Voice class.

Spiritual Groups

If you benefit from the experience of spirituality, and I find that most people, whose minds are open to possibility do benefit - check out your group to see if there are any sessions dealing with fitness. The Unity groups I know have wonderful classes and meetings dealing with this. I attend the Unity in New York. I attended for many years when Eric Butterworth, who found the center in New York, was alive. Now Rev. Justin Epstein heads the Unity Center, and sometimes I attend Unity of NY, another New York Unity group. On the Jewish high holidays, in recent years I've been attending JTS, the Jewish Theological Seminary.

Products

I take no medications, although I would take medicine, at least for a short term if my doctor said it would be necessary for me to do so. Thankfully because of all the research I've done, I've restored my health and don't require medicines.

I do take supplements. They were listed in the section about my mini-Qs. Many of the products I use are made by "multilevel marketing" companies. I take these products because people I trust recommended them to me. I find that I don't stick with the business end for a long time – however this might be a good way for YOU to earn some money while getting and staying healthy.

Barbara Van Diest introduced me to them and she always proved trustworthy.

If what I earn helps to pay something for the products, I'm happy. You can find trainers at these well-reputed companies who could help you if you wanted to make a business out of them.

1. Products made by Isagenix International
    a. Their supplements, interior cleansing products, and nourishing products are well made and have helped me greatly.

       (Again, I advise you to know what foods may not benefit your blood type. I choose the flavors of shakes that don't have whey protein in them. My blood type is A positive, and whey is on the "avoid" list for my blood type. That doesn't mean it's not good; it's just not good for my blood type. The Isagenix whey is very well made and de-natured.)

    b. I also recommend their Rejuvity facial cleanser.

       Note: the products work for men and women!

    c. You can visit my Isagenix site to find out more about the products: http://www.bobbiehorowitz.isagenix.com/en-US/landing-pages/contact-me And you can find my contact information on my site :www.bobbiehorowitz.com

2. Products made by MAX International. My body now manufactures its own glutathione naturally! Glutathione is an incredible, natural healing agent. There are very few cases in which it shouldn't be used. I think that if I'd had it before I needed cancer surgery, I wouldn't have needed cancer surgery.

3. Skin Creams by Nerium. These are the latest skin products that have been introduced to me. I wish you could feel my skin now and before I began using it! They don't, as yet, have many products. They have a body cream, a facial night cream, and a day cream. What they have has done wonders

for my skin in the short while since I heard about them. While I don't do this as a business it benefits me because when you enroll just three customers who get products monthly you can get them for free. That's a good deal. You can find my contact information on my site if you want to speak with me and I can help you approach 3 people to buy the product.

I invite you to read my "Reveal the Star You Truly Are" blog, which you can find on my Healthy, Wealthy & Wow! website by going to www.bobbiehorowitz.com. Select the tab Blog

You'll see additional unsolicited recommendations and learn about the above recommendations.

You'll find out about the products and professionals I mentioned and about additional products and professionals who provide services that can help you. You may want to contact them, and if you're not from their area, they may be able to recommend a practitioner in their field who works in your area. You'll be able to link to their websites whenever possible. New recommendations are added as I find new things t recommend.

Please note that I've asked for permission to list the companies and people listed on my site. They have not solicited me.

You'll get lots of free information and info about what's coming up!

- Get a free Image Tip every month on my site.
- Get tons of free information in the descriptions of the services I offer. (I've been told I have a hard time not giving away the store!)
- Free blog: Subscribe to my clear, short, to-the-point, and free blog, and you'll continually get many free image and fitness tips.

- You'll get to see what's coming up and check out upcoming seminars: Dress To Get "Yes!"—Color Psychology.

If any of these interest you, please tell your company, church group, social group, etc. about them, and I can fly to your town.

CHAPTER 17

Reveal the Star You Truly Are!

Do it your way! Have fun doing it!

This chapter can be short, yet it can take a lifetime to incorporate what I'm hopefully communicating. Some people never get there. I'm so glad that you will. If you follow the path of getting your physical self into the best shape it can be and keep it in it's best possible condition, you're well on your way to learning the most important thing I think anyone can learn. As I said before in this book, I'm continually working on it myself.

What am I referring to as the most important thing?

Learn to love yourself. It's totally worth your time!

When you love yourself, the actions you choose will help others to love themselves. Now that you're learning to love your body (the vehicle you were given to travel Earth in), you'll have one more reason to acknowledge the miracle you are. By the way, I don't define miracle to mean something unworldly. I believe that miracle is simply "what is." We just have to chip away what isn't the miracle.

Note: I mentioned Professor Milton R. Konvitz in my acknowledgments. I saw a note that I wrote during a lecture in his course, The Development of American Ideals. One of the topics covered was the manner in which the Judeo-Christian part of the American heritage influenced the development of our country. (I have a feeling the other religions have writings on this topic too.) In my notes, I wrote that he stated the most important commandment in terms of humans living together in harmony was the second commandment: "Love your neighbor as you love yourself." Then he said, "I bet if you look around you, you'll notice that everyone loves their neighbor just the way they love themselves!" I wouldn't have had the wisdom to make that up at that time, so he must have said it. I didn't fully get the importance of it until I reached my mid-sixties.

Think about that! You can chip away all that isn't truly you and *allow the star you truly are to shine.*

About Bobbie Horowitz

At age sixty-two, when most people are winding down, Bobbie Horowitz, songwriter, theatrical producer, and image consultant, became passionate about attaining and maintaining great health, looks, and vitality. In truth, necessity gave her no option! She wanted to keep living life to the fullest! After gaining forty-three pounds and developing painful osteoarthritis, a droopy neck, and cancer, she decided she'd better get back to her true self. Now - she's trim, her skin is smooth, and she has zero pain! Plus, she has fun staying this way—and she has stayed this way for well over thirteen years now! She feels blessed to have seemingly channeled a way that works for her and fits into her lifestyle … and she's thrilled that she can teach people to design their way, a way that fits into their lifestyle, using the mini-Q concept. The simple secrets are in this book, and she conducts workshops, should you wish one.

She was president of her high school, graduated first in her class from Cornell University's ILR School, and was certified in secondary education at Columbia University. She enjoyed working in her family's labor law firm for ten years, but when her son entered school, she had to fulfill her passion for theater. She studied with Stella Adler, Lee Strasberg, and Gene Frankel in their Master Class programs and appeared in over thirty-five NYC and regional productions. She won the Manhattan Association of Cabarets & Clubs Award as half of the songwriting/performing team Horowitz

& Spector and still writes songs on her own and with writers like David Friedman, John Meyer and Bill Zeffiro.

While acting, she was often asked to produce shows and also to create star-studded events at clubs like Studio 54 and Magique, including the "First Soap Opera Day" party along with Mayor Koch's office. It kept two soaps, employing many actors, in NYC. As Manhattan director of the Cystic Fibrosis Foundation, she coproduced the Farewell to Bowie Kuhn Dinner. She produced *The Betrayal of Nora Blake* in London after completing the Broadway League's fourteen-week CTI course at age fifty-seven. It won twelve out of twelve rave reviews and was then voted Best Musical in Florida. She was executive producer of the 1999 and 2000 Drama Desk Awards and associate producer of the 2001 awards presentation.

In her sixties, she founded the Times Square Group, an arts-in-education company.

In over twenty-five years of image consulting, she's served as VP of education for the tri-state chapter of AICI, has taught classes at many colleges and acting schools, has served private clients, has written articles, and has been quoted as an expert in *Seventeen* magazine.

By her mid-sixties, Bobbie finally realized that the things she'd done, though varied, have all been directed toward one mission: to see to it that everyone loves themselves! Bobbie believes that when the day everyone loves him/herself comes about – we can have peace on this planet.

NOTE: If you'd like to know when Bobbie is presenting workshops, seminars and webinars go to her site: www. bobbiehorowitz.com You can contact her from the site.

NOTE: If you enjoy a good time listening to music or going to theater – check Bobbie's performance, etc. schedule by clicking on the tab Songwriter/Performer

and you'll automatically be taken to her <u>www.</u>
<u>bobbiehorowitzproductions.com</u> site.

Some of Bobbie's shows are live streamed so you can
see them wherever you live. The link will be given on
the announcement of the show.

CPSIA information can be obtained
at www.ICGtesting.com
Printed in the USA
FFOW05n0941020915